Easy Planning in Elective Primary Orthopedic Procedures

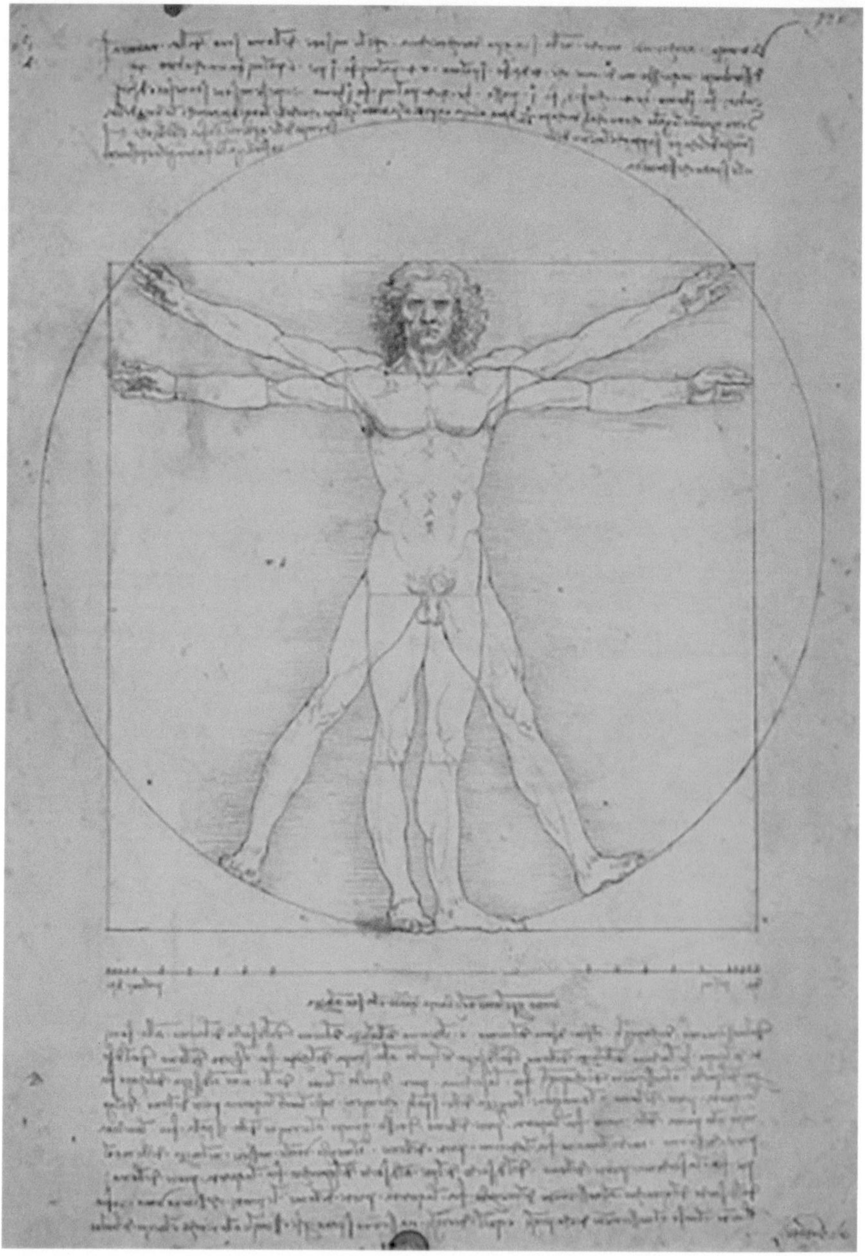

The Vitruvian Man by Leonardo da Vinci, By permission of the Italian Ministry of Culture

Giulio Maria Marcheggiani Muccioli
Gazi Huri • Alberto Grassi
Stefano Zaffagnini
Editors

Easy Planning in Elective Primary Orthopedic Procedures

Springer

Editors
Giulio Maria Marcheggiani Muccioli
Istituto Ortopedico Rizzoli
University of Bologna
Bologna, Italy

Gazi Huri
Orthopaedics and Traumatology Dept.
Hacettepe University School of Medicine
Ankara, Türkiye

Alberto Grassi
Istituto Ortopedico Rizzoli
University of Bologna
Bologna, Italy

Stefano Zaffagnini
Istituto Ortopedico Rizzoli
University of Bologna
Bologna, Italy

ISBN 978-3-031-77008-1 ISBN 978-3-031-77006-7 (eBook)
https://doi.org/10.1007/978-3-031-77006-7

This Springer imprint is published by the registered company Springer Nature Switzerland AG
The registered company address is: Gewerbestrasse 11, 6330 Cham, Switzerland

To the orthopedic residents of Istituto Ortopedico Rizzoli and all the orthopedic residents of the world: you are always an inspiration to fight for excellence.

Giulio Maria Marcheggiani Muccioli, MD, PhD, Associate Professor

I dedicate this book to those who lost their lives in the earthquake on February 6, 2023, and to my beautiful hometown, Antakya.

Gazi Huri, MD, PhD, Full Professor

I wish to thank every colleague, clinician, trainee, and patient who gives me the motivation to teach and train new generations of orthopedic surgeons.

A special thanks to my wife Andrea, for the hard task of supporting me every day in pursuing my passion.

Alberto Grassi, MD, PhD, Associate Professor

To all the people who work with me and to all the residents at the orthopedic school of the University of Bologna… hard work, planning and deep understanding of surgical technique are the keys of success.

Stefano Zaffagnini, MD, PhD, Full Professor and Chair

Senior Editor's Preface

The field of orthopedic surgery is highly competitive, particularly for orthopedic residents. I am delighted to present this book as it provides a unique opportunity for orthopedic and trauma surgery trainees to comprehend the significance of preoperative planning.

This comprehensive guide addresses the essential knowledge that orthopedic residents should acquire before stepping into the operating room. Each chapter meticulously covers the fundamentals of the most common elective orthopedic procedures, offering a valuable resource for those preparing to embark on their surgical careers.

I am particularly content with this book, anticipating that it will play a crucial role in aiding trainees to enhance their understanding and proficiency in the field. The emphasis on the importance of preoperative planning is a distinctive feature that sets this book apart, providing readers with insights that are instrumental in achieving optimal outcomes in surgical interventions.

I extend my heartfelt gratitude to all the colleagues who contributed to this project, demonstrating outstanding dedication and expertise. Special thanks also go to the other editors for extending the invitation to participate in this remarkable endeavor. This collaborative effort has truly resulted in a remarkable work that I believe will make a meaningful impact on the education and practice of orthopedic surgery.

Prof. Stefano Zaffagnini

Editor's Preface

This is a book for people who start their journey in the field of orthopedic surgery. It is not intended to be a manual of surgery, but a concise reference guide to reduce errors in the operating room.

Surgery is like life. It is not possible to experience it without making mistakes.

Modern surgery is built on the mistakes of the past. Planning is a good instrument to reduce errors, avoid mistakes of the past and be prepared to become a surgeon.

The only real mistake is the one from which we learn nothing. (Henry Ford)

This book is dedicated to my family, the love of my life and the source of my energy.

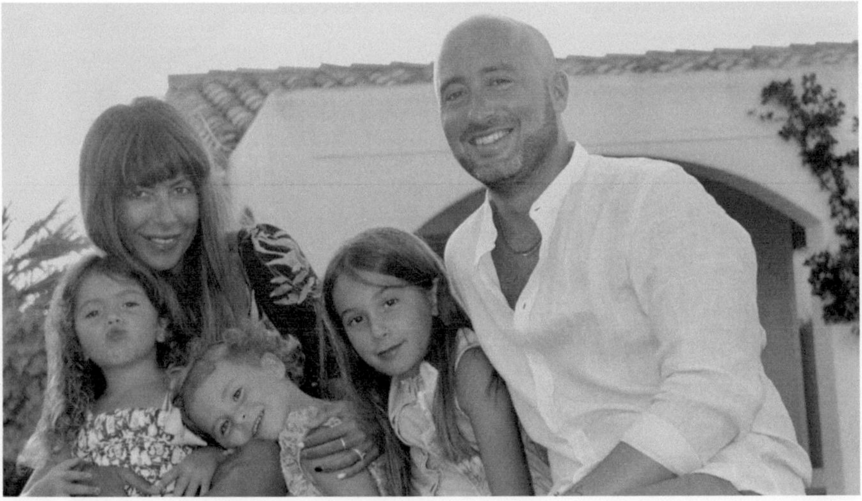

Prof. Giulio Maria Marcheggiani Muccioli

Acknowledgments

We thank all the nurses and all the staff of our hospitals for their help and their patience during all these years of surgery together.

We thank our illustrators, Silvia Bassini and Maria Pia Cumani, for the wonderful work and for their crucial help in creating this manuscript.

Contents

Part I Shoulder Arthroplasty

1 Patient Position and General Setting in Shoulder Arthroplasty 3
A. Beydemir, G. Dursun, E. Ertekin, and G. Huri

2 Planning in Resurfacing (Stemless) Shoulder Arthroplasty 11
E. Özdemir, Y. Yiğit, U. Kanlıkaya, and G. Huri

3 Preoperative Planning in Anatomic Shoulder Arthroplasty 19
A. De Vita, R. Russo, and F. Familiari

4 RTSA for Primary Osteoarthritis: Preoperative Planning 33
M. Monetta, M. Riva, F. Tortorella, F. Coliva, M. Cavallo, and E. Guerra

Part II Elbow Arthroplasty

5 Patient Position and General Setting in Elbow Arthroplasty 53
F. Coliva, A. Sessa, M. Monetta, A. Ritali, G. Carbone, and E. Guerra

6 Planning in Total Elbow Arthroplasty 59
F. Tortorella, L. Ferra, A. Marinelli, C. Buondonno, M. Cavallo, and E. Guerra

7 Planning in Elbow Hemiarthroplasty 71
C. Buondonno, A. Marinelli, L. Ferra, M. Riva, A. Sessa, and E. Guerra

Part III Hip Arthroplasty

8 Patient Position and General Setting in Total Hip Arthroplasty 85
F. Raggi, T. Cerasoli, D. Alesi, Giulio Maria Marcheggiani Muccioli, M. Zaffagnini, E. Tassinari, and Stefano Zaffagnini

9 Preoperative Planning for Primary Total Hip Arthroplasty 97
F. Raggi, D. Alesi, M. Zaffagnini, M. Casali, Giulio Maria Marcheggiani Muccioli, M. Romagnoli, and Stefano Zaffagnini

10 Planning in Robotic-Assisted Total Hip Arthroplasty 105
Sonia K. Chandi, Simarjeet Puri, Colin C. Neitzke, Eytan M. Debbi, and Brian P. Chalmers

Part IV Osteotomy Around the Hip in Adults

11 Planning of Femoral Osteotomy for Hip Dysplasia 119
Yutaka Inaba, Taro Tezuka, and Yukihide Minoda

Part V Knee Arthroplasty

12 Patient Position and General Setting in Knee Arthroplasty 129
V. G. Rinaldi, E. Cammisa, I. Sassoli, M. La Verde, A. Fogacci, and Giulio Maria Marcheggiani Muccioli

13 Planning in Unicompartmental (Medial, Lateral, and Patellofemoral) Knee Artroplasty 135
S. Fratini, I. Sassoli, A. Fogacci, M. P. Neri, M. Lo Presti, and Giulio Maria Marcheggiani Muccioli

14 Preoperative Planning for Primary Total Knee Arthroplasty (Mechanical, Anatomic, and Kinematic Alignment) 145
D. Alesi, B. Al-Zubi, S. Fratini, E. Cammisa, M. La Verde, and Giulio Maria Marcheggiani Muccioli

15 Preoperative Planning in Robotic-Assisted Knee Arthroplasty 159
Heather J. Roberts and Nicholas A. Bedard

Part VI Osteotomy Around the Knee

16 Patient Position and General Setting in Osteotomy Around the Knee 171
A. Grassi, E. Altovino, G. A. Lucidi, N. Maitan, M. Viotto, and Stefano Zaffagnini

17 Planning in High Tibial Osteotomy for Varus Knee 179
A. Grassi, V. Davidoni, G. Dal Fabbro, P. Agostinone, and Stefano Zaffagnini

18 Planning in Distal Femoral Osteotomy for Valgus Knee 189
A. Grassi, P. Agostinone, G. Dal Fabbro, G. A. Lucidi, A. Pagano, and Stefano Zaffagnini

Part VII Ankle Arthroplasty

19 Patient Positioning and Planning in Total Ankle Replacement Through Anterior and Lateral Approach 199
S. Caravelli, M. Viotto, G. Puccetti, A. Baiardi, M. Di Ponte, B. Khateeb, and M. Mosca

Part VIII Common Osteotomy Around Foot and Ankle in Adults

20 Planning in Common Osteotomy Around Foot and Ankle in Adults 209
S. Caravelli, M. Viotto, M. Di Ponte, B. Khateeb, E. Vocale, G. Gardini, and M. Mosca

Part I

Shoulder Arthroplasty

G. Huri

1 Patient Position and General Setting in Shoulder Arthroplasty

A. Beydemir, G. Dursun, E. Ertekin, and G. Huri

1.1 Introduction

Pain and limitation of range of motion may occur in the shoulder joint as a result of osteoarthritis, rheumatoid arthritis, trauma, avascular necrosis, rotator cuff arthropathy, infection, and arthropathy due to neurological diseases [1]. Shoulder arthroplasty is indicated to relieve pain and restore shoulder joint function in patients who do not respond to conservative treatment [2]. With the increasing life expectancy of the patients, the amount of shoulder arthroplasty performed today is gradually increasing [3]. Appropriate patient positioning and a comprehensive general setting are vital for performing shoulder arthroplasty effectively and with the least possible complications.

This chapter aims to emphasize the importance of patient positioning and general setting in shoulder arthroplasty and to draw attention to important points.

1.2 Anesthesia

Shoulder arthroplasty can be performed under general anesthesia, regional anesthesia (e.g., interscalene nerve block), or a combination of them. General anesthesia enhances muscle relaxation improving exposure of the glenoid, which is a key

A. Beydemir · G. Dursun · E. Ertekin
Department of Orthopaedic and Traumatology, Hacettepe University, Ankara, Turkey

G. Huri (✉)
Department of Orthopaedic and Traumatology, Hacettepe University, Ankara, Turkey

Aspetar FIFA Center of Excellence, Orthopaedcis and Sports Medicine Hospital, Doha, Qatar
e-mail: gazi.huri@hacettepe.edu.tr

G. M. Marcheggiani Muccioli et al. (eds.), *Easy Planning in Elective Primary Orthopedic Procedures*, https://doi.org/10.1007/978-3-031-77006-7_1

factor in the success of shoulder replacement surgery [4]. The advantages of regional anesthesia include better intraoperative and postoperative pain control, reduced postoperative opioid use, shorter recovery time, and a decreased length of hospital stay [5, 6]. One of the most critical complications of beach chair position under general anesthesia is cerebral hypoperfusion. Studies have reported a decrease in cerebral perfusion pressure in patients placed in the beach chair position under general anesthesia [7]. Although it is rare, devastating neurological events related to cerebral hypoperfusion, such as ischemic stroke and spinal cord injury, have been reported in the literature [8–10]. Since interscalene nerve block with sedation may help prevent cerebral hypoperfusion, regional anesthesia is recommended whenever possible [11, 12].

1.3 Patient Positioning

Proper patient positioning for shoulder arthroplasty will reduce potential complications and facilitate the surgical intervention. The following two matters are critical in the patient positioning: adequate humerus exposure, which requires extension, adduction, and external rotation, and optimal glenoid exposure, which must face the operator as far as possible [13]. Since the shoulder should be positioned in the extension, adduction, and external rotation during the placement of the humeral component and the reaming of the humeral canal, care should be taken not to interfere with the edge of the operating table. The patient is placed in the beach chair position. Skyhar et al. first described its use in shoulder arthroscopy in 1988 [14]. The patient is placed supine on the operating table, with the head secured in a positioner. The operating table is first reflexed to achieve 30°–40° of hip flexion, and the operating table is then placed in a slightly "Trendelenburg position" to prevent the patient from sliding down (Fig. 1.1) The patient's knees are flexed 30° to relieve sciatic nerve tension and reduce popliteal fossa pressure. In addition, pads should be

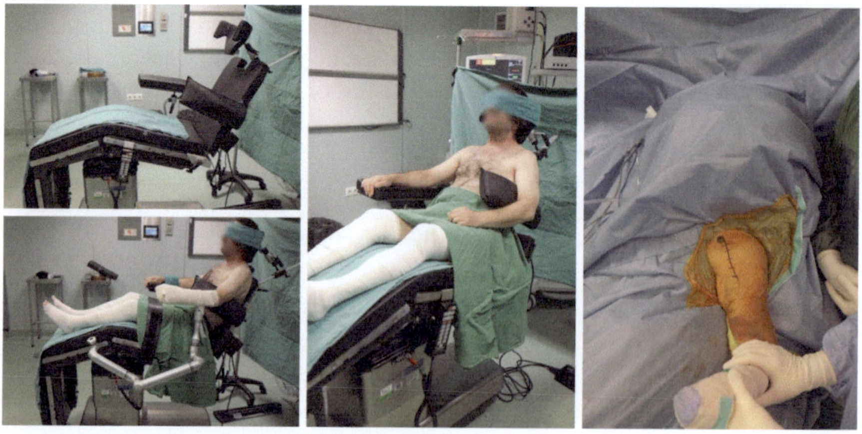

Fig. 1.1 Patient position and final surgical draping

placed on the knees to prevent peroneal nerve neuropraxia [15]. An elastic compression bandage is applied to the patient's legs above the knees for deep vein thrombosis prophylaxis. A strap should be placed as a seat belt over the patient's thighs. Lastly, the back of the operating table is elevated at 60°. To allow anterior dislocation of the humerus during the procedure, the ipsilateral back third of the table is removed, exposing the posterior aspect of the shoulder. The contralateral arm is placed on an arm support, and a pad is placed under the elbow to prevent ulnar nerve neuropraxia.

After the beach chair position is provided, the position of the patient's head and neck should be checked to ensure neutral alignment (Fig. 1.1). Once the head and neck position is acceptable, the patient's head is secured to the head positioner with a head restraint across the patient's forehead and under the chin to assure stability [16].

1.4 Surgical Preparation and Draping

Skin preparation should begin one day before the operation to reduce surgical site infection and avoid skin irritation. Patients are advised to shave their body, including the arm's shoulder girdle, axilla, and elbow. The most common cause of periprosthetic joint infection after shoulder arthroplasty is *Propionibacterium acnes*. Other common agents are *Staphylococcus aureus*, *Staphylococcus epidermidis*, and coagulase-negative Staphylococci [17, 18].

Prophylactic antibiotics are considered the standard of care in preventing periprosthetic joint infection and should be administrated 30 min before the skin incision [19]. Antibiotic prophylaxis with cefazolin is associated with a significantly lower rate of periprosthetic joint infection compared with other alternative regimens (e.g., vancomycin, clindamycin, and others) [20].

After the patient is positioned on the operating table, the skin of the shoulder girdle is prepared, and the entire upper extremity (including the hand) is precleaned with isopropyl alcohol. A surgical scrub is then applied to the same areas. The scrub is performed with a 4% chlorhexidine gluconate solution, or povidone-iodine (Betadine) 10% solution if the patient is allergic to chlorhexidine. After the surgical area is dried with sterile towels, the entire upper extremity (including the hand) is painted with 4% chlorhexidine gluconate solution, starting around the estimated incision line and expanding with circular movements, medially to the midsternal line, inferiorly to the nipple, and proximal to the mandible. The axilla is painted last.

The first aim of draping the surgical patient is to isolate the surgical site from the other nonsterile areas to reduce the risk of surgical site infection. Draping begins with an assistant draping the impermeable stockinet from the hand over the elbow. In extensile approaches, the impermeable stockinet can extend from the hand to the forearm. Then stockinet is covered and secured with and disposable elastic wrap. Since the drape will not adhere to the skin when wet, the shoulder area should be dried with a sterile towel before draping. An impermeable reinforced "U" drape is placed inferiorly and superiorly; finally, a Betadine-impregnated adhesive drape is applied to cover the skin thoroughly (Fig. 1.1).

1.5 Operating Room Layout

The operating room, where shoulder arthroplasty is performed, should preferably be spacious to store the implant sets, move them quickly, and minimize staff traffic. The operating room has two doors. The main door is where the patient enters the room and stays closed during the surgery to minimize staff traffic. The second door opens to the sterilization area.

Anesthesia equipment is located at the head of the patient next to the anesthesiologist; the power source, cautery generator, and tubing for suction are located at the nonoperative side of the patient behind the second assistant. In the operating room, two Mayo stands are located behind the foot of the patient. One of the Mayo stands has mobile shelving units containing all standard sets of implants, while the other has mobile shelving units containing specific prosthetic equipment. The operating table is placed directly under the operating lights. Proper lighting and the angle of incidence of the light on the surgical site are critical for the proper performance of shoulder arthroplasty. The main light is positioned above the left shoulder of the dominant right-hand surgeon, and the secondary light is on the right shoulder of the surgeon but more on the head of the patient. A computer may be available to review preoperative digital imaging in the operating room.

1.6 Surgical Team Layout

Figure A shows the position of each member of the staff. The anesthesiologist is located at the head of the operating table. The surgeon operating the patient stands facing the patient's axilla to provide a better perspective (Fig. 1.2). The first assistant stands behind the surgical shoulder next to the operating surgeon. If a second assistant is present in the operating room, this assistant stands on the nonoperative side of the operating table. The second assistant provides retraction from the nonoperative side of the operating table. In this way, there is no crowd around the surgeon, and if there is an observer in the room, this ensures that the observers have an unhindered view of the procedure. The nurse stands on the nonoperative side of the patient next to the second assistant (Fig. 1.2).

1.7 Surgical Instrumentation

Figure 1.3 shows the arrangement of the first Mayo stand, where the most commonly used surgical instruments were placed to perform a shoulder arthroplasty.

The second Mayo stand with special prosthetic instrument humeral and glenoid sets should also be available in the operating room.

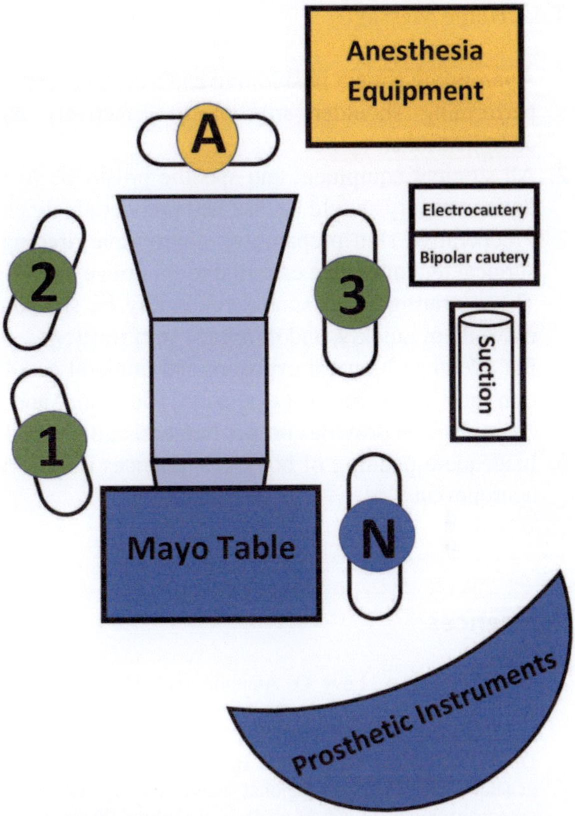

Fig. 1.2 Surgical team and operating room layout

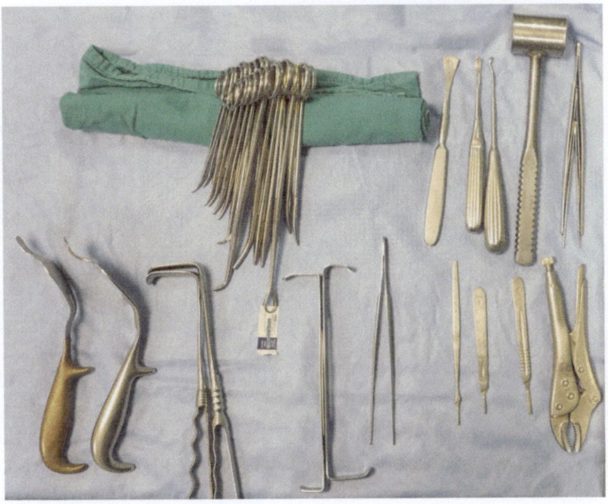

Fig. 1.3 Arrangement of surgical instruments

Take Home Messages

1. Appropriate patient positioning and a comprehensive general setting are vital for performing shoulder arthroplasty effectively and with the least possible complications.
2. All surgical equipment and specific prosthetic instrumentation sets to be used during surgery should be checked preoperatively and completed during surgery.
3. Preoperative skin preparation, appropriate draping, and painting according to surgical technique are essential to minimize the risk of postoperative infection.
4. The operating room should preferably be spacious to store the implant sets, move them quickly, and minimize staff traffic.
5. For adequate humeral exposure and humeral canal reaming, the patient's position must allow for arm extension, adduction, and external rotation. The beach chair position provides proper humeral and glenoid exposure.
6. Inadequate padding of bony prominences should be avoided as this may cause neuropraxia.

References

1. Oren T, Ehud A, Levy O. Anatomic shoulder arthroplasty. In: Huri G, Paschos N, editors. The shoulder, Orthopaedic study guide series. Cham: Springer; 2017. https://doi.org/10.1007/978-3-319-51979-1_21.
2. Ding DY, Mahure SA, Mollon B, Shamah SD, Zuckerman JD, Kwon YW. Comparison of general versus isolated regional anesthesia in total shoulder arthroplasty: a retrospective propensity-matched cohort analysis. J Orthop. 2017;14(4):417–24. https://doi.org/10.1016/j.jor.2017.07.002. PMID: 28794581; PMCID: PMC5537444.
3. Farley KX, Wilson JM, Kumar A, Gottschalk MB, Daly C, Sanchez-Sotelo J, Wagner ER. Prevalence of shoulder arthroplasty in the United States and the increasing burden of revision shoulder arthroplasty. JB JS Open Access. 2021;6(3):e20.00156. https://doi.org/10.2106/JBJS.OA.20.00156. PMID: 34278185; PMCID: PMC8280071.
4. Boin MA, Mehta D, Dankert J, Umeh UO, Zuckerman JD, Virk MS. Anesthesia in total shoulder arthroplasty: a systematic review and meta-analysis. JBJS Rev. 2021;9(11) https://doi.org/10.2106/JBJS.RVW.21.00115.
5. Stundner O, Rasul R, Chiu YL, Sun X, Mazumdar M, Brummett CM, Ortmaier R, Memtsoudis SG. Peripheral nerve blocks in shoulder arthroplasty: how do they influence complications and length of stay. Clin Orthop Relat Res. 2014;472(5):1482–8.
6. Lee HY, Kim SH, So KY, Kim DJ. Effects of interscalene brachial plexus block to intra-operative hemodynamics and postoperative pain for arthroscopic shoulder surgery. Korean J Anesthesiol. 2012;62:30–4.
7. Soeding PF, Wang J, Hoy G, Jarman P, Phillips H, Marks P, Royse C. The effect of the sitting upright or 'beachchair' position on cerebral blood flow during anaesthesia for shoulder surgery. Anaesth Intensive Care. 2011;39(3):440–8. https://doi.org/10.1177/0310057X1103900315. PMID: 21675064.
8. Pohl A, Cullen DJ. Cerebral ischemia during shoulder surgery in the upright position: a case series. J Clin Anesth. 2005;17(6):463–9. https://doi.org/10.1016/j.jclinane.2004.09.012. PMID: 16171668.

9. Koga T, Miyao M, Sato M, Hirota K, Kakuyama M, Tanabe H, Fukuda K. Pituitary apoplexy during general anesthesia in beach chair position for shoulder joint arthroplasty. J Anesth. 2010;24(3):476–8. https://doi.org/10.1007/s00540-010-0929-y. Epub 2010 Mar 26. PMID: 20339880.
10. Papadonikolakis A, Wiesler ER, Olympio MA, Poehling GG. Avoiding catastrophic complications of stroke and death related to shoulder surgery in the sitting position. Arthroscopy. 2008;24(4):481–2. https://doi.org/10.1016/j.arthro.2008.02.005. PMID: 18375282.
11. Koh JL, Levin SD, Chehab EL, Murphy GS. Neer Award 2012: cerebral oxygenation in the beach chair position: a prospective study on the effect of general anesthesia compared with regional anesthesia and sedation. J Shoulder Elb Surg. 2013;22(10):1325–31. https://doi.org/10.1016/j.jse.2013.01.035. Epub 2013 Apr 6. PMID: 23571083.
12. Kotha R, Orebaugh SL. Shoulder surgery in the beach chair position: current anesthetic concepts and controversies in hemodynamic management and cerebral perfusion. Adv Anesth. 2014;32(1):pxiii–xviii.
13. Gadea F, Bouju Y, Berhouet J, Bacle G, Favard L. Deltopectoral approach for shoulder arthroplasty: anatomic basis. Int Orthop. 2015;39(2):215–25. https://doi.org/10.1007/s00264-014-2654-x. Epub 2015 Jan 16. PMID: 25592830.
14. Skyhar MJ, Altchek DW, Warren RF, Wickiewicz TL, O'Brien SJ. Shoulder arthroscopy with the patient in the beach-chair position. Arthroscopy. 1988;4(4):256–9. https://doi.org/10.1016/s0749-8063(88)80040-9. PMID: 3233114.
15. Öztürk Ö, Ergün S, Akgün U. Positioning, anesthesia, and analgesia in shoulder surgery. In: Huri G, Özkan M, Bilsel K, editors. Fundamentals of the shoulder. Cham: Springer; 2022. https://doi.org/10.1007/978-3-030-94702-6_15.
16. Van Tongel A, Hardeman F, Karelse A, de Wilde L. Positioning of the patient during shoulder surgery: an inexpensive, safe and easy technique. Eur J Orthop Surg Traumatol. 2013;23(1):115–7. https://doi.org/10.1007/s00590-011-0935-2. Epub 2011 Dec 31. PMID: 23412417.
17. Egglestone A, Ingoe H, Rees J, Thomas M, Jeavons R, Rangan A. Scoping review: diagnosis and management of periprosthetic joint infection in shoulder arthroplasty. Shoulder Elbow. 2019;11:167–81. https://doi.org/10.1177/1758573218779076.
18. Saltzman MD, Marecek GS, Edwards SL, Kalainov DM. Infection after shoulder surgery. J Am Acad Orthop Surg. 2011;19:208–18.
19. Boyle KK, Duquin TR. Antibiotic prophylaxis and prevention of surgical site infection in shoulder and elbow surgery. Orthop Clin North Am. 2018;49:241–56. https://doi.org/10.1016/j.ocl.2017.11.011.
20. Marigi EM, Bartels DW, Yoon JH, Sperling JW, Sanchez-Sotelo J. Antibiotic prophylaxis with cefazolin is associated with lower shoulder periprosthetic joint infection rates than non-cefazolin alternatives. J Bone Joint Surg Am. 2022;104(10):872–80. https://doi.org/10.2106/JBJS.21.00445. Epub 2022 Feb 21. PMID:35188900.

Planning in Resurfacing (Stemless) Shoulder Arthroplasty

2

E. Özdemir, Y. Yiğit, U. Kanlıkaya, and G. Huri

2.1 Introduction

The number of patients undergoing total shoulder arthroplasty (TSA) and reverse shoulder arthroplasty (RTSA) has significally increased in the last decade [1]. RTSA has gained more popularity accounting for the 33% of all shoulder arthroplasties, while TSA and hemiarthroplasty take 44% and 23%, respectively [2]. Along with the rapid increase in the incidence of shoulder arthroplasties, implant designs have evolved rapidly, including the development of stemless humeral components.

The newly introduced stemless shoulder arthroplasty design aims to preserve the humeral intramedullary canal and relies on cementless metaphyseal fixation in the proximal humerus. The fixation of the stemless component to the proximal humerus shares the same bone ingrowth philosophy of various implant designs, either via a coating or a specific material at the bone–implant interface. The rationale for developing stemless shoulder arthroplasty is to reduce stem-related complications. The theoretical advantages of stemless arthroplasty include the preservation of bone stock in the proximal humerus, the elimination of broaching (thereby reducing the risk of periprosthetic fractures), the reduction of stress shielding and stress riser points around the proximal humerus, easier reconstruction of the proximal humerus in case of malunion, less complex revision surgeries due to preserved bone stock, and reduced intraoperative bleeding and surgical time [3]. Because stemless shoulder arthroplasty does not need intramedullary preparation, removing the prior humerus plating or elbow arthroplasty is unnecessary. Given these potential advantages of stemless shoulder arthroplasty, its incidence is expected to grow in the near future [4].

E. Özdemir · Y. Yiğit · U. Kanlıkaya · G. Huri (✉)
Department of Orthopaedic and Traumatology, Hacettepe University, Ankara, Turkey

Aspetar FIFA Center of Excellence, Orthopaedcis and Sports Medicine Hospital, Doha, Qatar
e-mail: gazi.huri@hacettepe.edu.tr

G. M. Marcheggiani Muccioli et al. (eds.), *Easy Planning in Elective Primary Orthopedic Procedures*, https://doi.org/10.1007/978-3-031-77006-7_2

However, stemless shoulder arthroplasty has potential disadvantages. The most significant is component loosening before the accomplishment of bony ingrowth. The bony ingrowth is strongly related to the proximal humerus bone stock. In a lesser tuberosity osteotomy, it is challenging to provide fixation after placement of the stemless humerus designs. Nevertheless, this theoretical disadvantage is solved by surgical techniques and materials developments, including suture anchors, transosseous tunnels, and direct tendon-to-tendon repair [5]. Although stemless humeral component theoretically decreases periprosthetic fracture risk, there is still a risk of lateral cortex fracture during implantation. Controlling the inclination of the implant is more complicated than in stemmed shoulder arthroplasty, and it may affect the outcomes, particularly in RTSA.

2.2 Indications

Primary and secondary glenohumeral arthritis is the most common indication for stemless shoulder arthroplasty [6]. Stemless arthroplasty has been used for rheumatoid arthritis and other inflammatory arthritis, rotator cuff tear arthropathy, posttraumatic arthritis, postinfectious arthritis, and secondary arthritis due to glenoid dysplasia. The indications of stemless shoulder arthroplasty are similar to those for stemmed shoulder arthroplasties, as stemless humeral component designs are available for TSA, RTSA, and HA (Fig. 2.1).

The success of stemless arthroplasty is highly associated with appropriate diagnosis and restoration of native proximal humerus anatomy. The anatomic version of the humeral head depends on the individual and can range from 5° of anteversion to 55° of retroversion [7]. Any alteration in offset, inclination, or version, during the

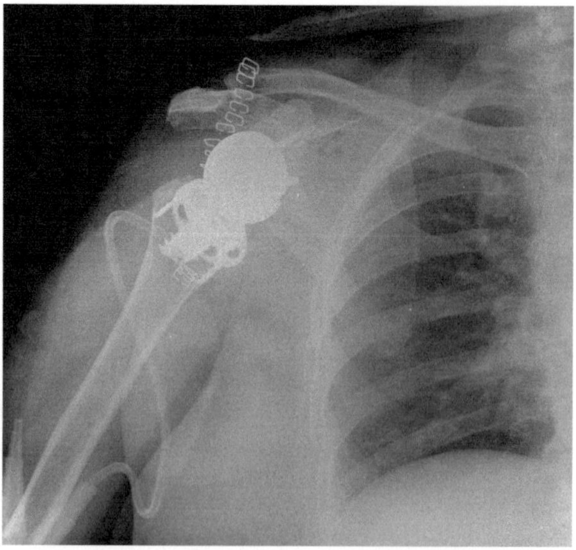

Fig. 2.1 A stemless reverse total shoulder arthroplasty design preserving the proximal humerus bone stock and humerus intramedullary canal

restoration of native anatomy can affect shoulder biomechanics and interfere with the surgical outcome.

Proximal humerus bone stock is essential in selecting the appropriate humeral component [8]. Stemless shoulder arthroplasty requires good bone quality to achieve press-fit metaphyseal fixation. The intraoperative "thumb test" is a subjective method for the assessment of bone quality in the proximal humerus. Although the "thumb test" is a common technique, the intraoperative conversion from a stemless shoulder system to a stemmed system occurs in only 1% of cases [9]. In addition, a change in decision during surgery can increase surgical time and cost. Therefore, the deltoid tuberosity index (DTI) and the Hounsfield units (HU) of the proximal humerus should be considered during preoperative decision-making for an appropriate humeral stem. Levin et al. proposed that preoperative DTI has a good predictive ability, while preoperative HU has an excellent predictive ability in categorizing patients as appropriate for stemless TSA [10].

2.3 Contraindications

There are some absolute contraindications for stemless shoulder arthroplasty. General contraindication for a shoulder arthroplasty includes active infection and paralysis of the deltoid and rotator cuff muscles. The main contraindication for stemless shoulder arthroplasty is the absence of adequate bone stock for metaphyseal fixation. Acute fractures at the proximal humerus are also contraindications for stemless shoulder arthroplasty [11].

Further contraindications that can reduce bone stock at the proximal humerus include severe rheumatoid arthritis with large subchondral cysts, large humeral head bony defects, poor humeral head bone quality that cannot resist forces after implantation, avascular necrosis involving more than 40% of the humeral head, and malignancies around the proximal humerus.

2.4 Preoperative Radiographic Evaluation

A good preoperative radiographic evaluation allows the surgeon to predict component sizes of the glenoid component, humeral head, and stem preference, and it also can avoid intraoperative complications and improve postoperative outcomes and patient satisfaction.

Patients with primary glenohumeral osteoarthritis often have glenoid retroversion due to posterior glenoid rim erosions or preexisting glenoid dysplasia [12]. Postoperative glenoid component retroversion is associated with an increased rate of radiolucency, component loosening, humeral head dislocation, and glenoid wear. In order to restore normal glenohumeral joint biomechanics after arthroplasty, surgical correction to a neutral version via eccentric anterior glenoid reaming is performed in mild to moderate cases. In more severe cases of glenoid retroversion (>20 degrees), bone grafting may be used [13].

True anteroposterior (AP), scapular Y, and axillary shoulder radiographs are crucial for preoperative radiographic evaluation (Fig. 2.2); however, they have poor interobserver and intraobserver reproducibility and overestimate the degree of retroversion. Computed tomography (CT) has higher reproducibility than radiographs (Fig. 2.3) [14]. Friedman described the glenoid version on two-dimensional (2D) CT as the angle formed between a line drawn from the medial border of the scapula to the center of the glenoid and the line perpendicular to the face of the glenoid on the axial slice at or just below the tip of the coracoid of the scapula [15].

The Walch classification of glenoid morphology is assessed on axillary radiographs or axial CT images:

- Type A morphology is a centered humeral head with minor or major glenoid erosions.
- Type B morphology is a posteriorly subluxated humeral head with posterior joint space narrowing and osteophytes or posterior rim erosions and retroversion.
- Type C morphology is with glenoid retroversion of > 25°, which is the most severe form.

Magnetic resonance imaging (MRI) is currently being investigated as another tool for assessing glenoid retroversion. A preliminary study showed MRI to have higher interobserver and intraobserver variability and lower mean retroversion angles compared with axillary radiographs [13]. MRI has the additional benefit of preoperatively assessing the rotator cuff and adjacent soft tissues. The other factor that should be assessed before surgery is the integrity of the subscapularis tendon. Contracture or tear of the subscapularis tendon is associated with anterior instability if not corrected preoperatively [16].

Rotator cuff integrity is another factor that influences the type of shoulder arthroplasty. Narrowed acromiohumeral distance (<7 mm) with superior subluxation of

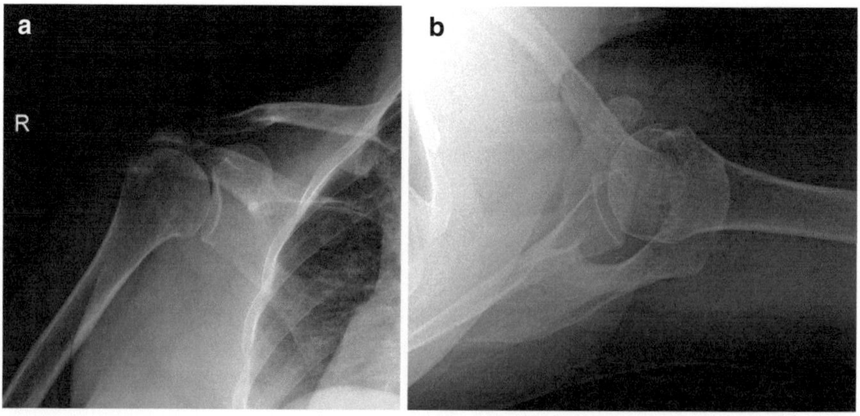

Fig. 2.2 (**a**) True anteroposterior shoulder radiograph of a patient showing rotator cuff tear arthropathy. (**b**) Axillary shoulder view shows no glenoid erosion

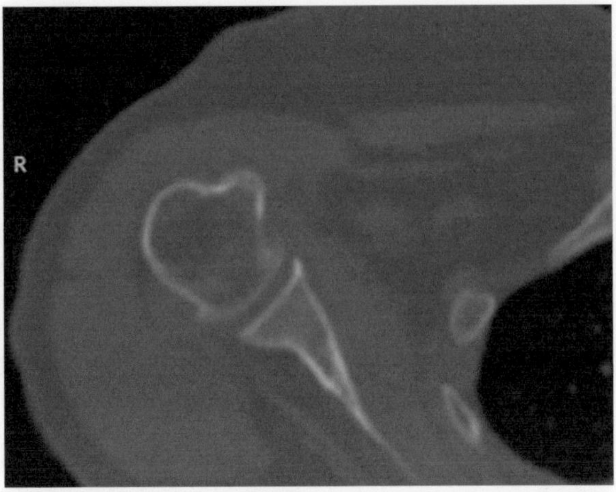

Fig. 2.3 A coronal computed tomography section provides better evaluation of glenoid erosion

the humeral head on AP radiographs correlates with full-thickness supraspinatus and infraspinatus tears and fatty muscle degeneration. Additionally, greater tuberosity sclerosis, irregularity and subchondral cysts, an exaggerated groove between the greater tuberosity and humeral articular surface, and "acetabularization" of the acromion (acromial undersurface remodeling) also suggest large rotator cuff tears [17]. Without definitive radiographic findings, MRI or ultrasound can be used to diagnose rotator cuff tears.

2.5 Recent Preoperative Digital Planning and Templating

Studies have recently shown three-dimensional (3D) CT is more accurate for planning (Fig. 2.4) shoulder arthroplasty and provides better positioning of the glenoid component than 2D CT scans through an improved understanding of both the pathologic and the premorbid glenoid joint line, version, and inclination compared to an ideal planned glenoid position [18].

3D templating software developed for shoulder arthroplasty allows virtual surgery to determine component size before surgery. Software programs based on preoperative CT scans allow the surgeon to perform cuts, visualize and test implant sizes, adjust version, and predict the virtual range of motion. This technology could potentially reduce factors that lead to the failure of TSA, such as glenoid loosening caused by both humeral and glenoid component malpositioning or incorrect sizing [19].

A study by Shukla et al. compared the measurements obtained using classic manual measuring techniques with those generated by automated image analysis software. Ninety-five 2D CT scans of shoulders with primary glenohumeral osteoarthritis were measured for version according to the Friedman method, inclination according to the Maurer method, and subluxation according to the Walch method. Average manual measurements included 13.8° version, 13.2° inclination, and 56.2%

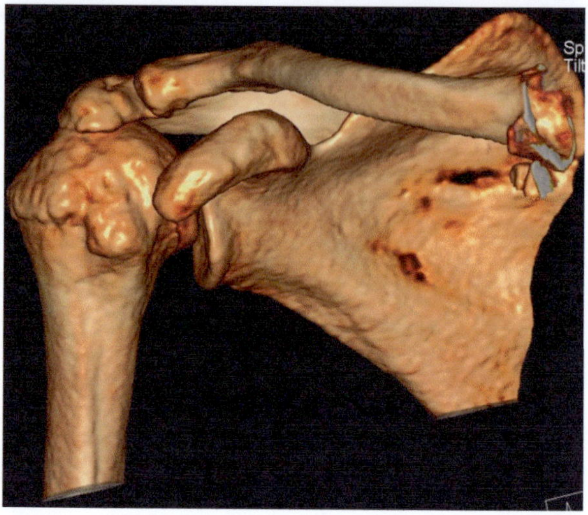

Fig. 2.4 A three-dimensional (3D) computed scan is more reliable for preoperative planning of shoulder arthroplasty

subluxation. Average image analysis software values included 17.4° version (3.5° difference), 9.2° inclination (3.9° difference), and 74.2% for subluxation (18% difference). The automated image analysis software provided relatively similar values to those obtained through manual measurement on 2D CT for the glenoid version and inclination [20].

A multicentered retrospective study was made in patients who undergo TSA utilizing 3D virtual planning technology that investigates preoperative templated implant size and its resemblance to actual implant size at the time of surgery. For stemless humeral components ($n = 87$) implanted, 98% matched the preoperative template within one size, with 79% exactly matched. This study demonstrates that preoperative 3D digital templating for anatomic TSAs can accurately predict the glenoid component size. The humeral component size prediction was very accurate with stemless implants. Preoperative 3D digital templating and computer simulation can potentially reduce overall TSA costs by managing the cost of implants and instrumentation, reducing inventory needs on an individual case basis, and helping to improve surgical efficiency [21].

Take Home Messages

1. Stemless shoulder arthroplasty relies mainly on cementless metaphyseal fixation and is created to avoid stem-related problems.
2. Compared to stemmed designs, the clinical outcome of stemless designs is equally good in the short- and medium-term follow-up.
3. The intraoperative fracture rate is lower in stemless designs than in stemmed designs, possibly due to the absence of intramedullary preparation and the stem implantation.
4. Preoperative radiographic evaluation is crucial for determining the appropriate humeral component.

5. The use of 3D software based on CT images has been reported to show promising results.
6. There are not enough long-term randomized trials to assess the superiority of stemless arthroplasty over stemmed shoulder arthroplasty.

References

1. Trofa D, Rajaee SS, Smith EL. Nationwide trends in total shoulder arthroplasty and hemiarthroplasty for osteoarthritis. Am J Orthop (Belle Mead NJ). 2014;43(4):166–72.
2. Schairer WW, Nwachukwu BU, Lyman S, Craig EV, Gulotta LV. National utilization of reverse total shoulder arthroplasty in the United States. J Shoulder Elb Surg. 2015;24(1):91–7.
3. Churchill RS, Athwal GS. Stemless shoulder arthroplasty-current results and designs. Curr Rev Musculoskelet Med. 2016;9(1):10–6.
4. Upfill-Brown A, Satariano N, Feeley B. Stemless shoulder arthroplasty: review of short and medium-term results. JSES Open Access. 2019;3(3):154–61.
5. Hawi N, Magosch P, Tauber M, Lichtenberg S, Habermeyer P. Nine-year outcome after anatomic stemless shoulder prosthesis: clinical and radiologic results. J Shoulder Elb Surg. 2017;26(9):1609–15.
6. Galhoum MS, Elsheikh AA, Wood A, Yin Q, Frostick SP. Anatomic and reverse stemless shoulder arthroplasty: functional and radiological evaluation. J Shoulder Elb Arthroplast. 2022;6:24715492221118765.
7. Thomas SR, Sforza G, Levy O, Copeland SA. Geometrical analysis of Copeland surface replacement shoulder arthroplasty in relation to normal anatomy. J Shoulder Elb Surg. 2005;14(2):186–92.
8. Churchill RS, Chuinard C, Wiater JM, Friedman R, Freehill M, Jacobson S, et al. Clinical and radiographic outcomes of the simpliciti canal-sparing shoulder arthroplasty system: a prospective two-year multicenter study. J Bone Joint Surg Am. 2016;98(7):552–60.
9. Liu EY, Kord D, Horner NS, Leroux T, Alolabi B, Khan M. Stemless anatomic total shoulder arthroplasty: a systematic review and meta-analysis. J Shoulder Elb Surg. 2020;29(9):1928–37.
10. Levin JM, Rodriguez K, Polascik BA, Zeng S, Warren E Jr, Rechenmacher A, et al. Simple preoperative radiographic and computed tomography measurements predict adequate bone quality for stemless total shoulder arthroplasty. J Shoulder Elb Surg. 2022;31(12):2481–7.
11. Willems JIP, Hoffmann J, Sierevelt IN, van den Bekerom MPJ, Alta TDW, van Noort A. Results of stemless shoulder arthroplasty: a systematic review and meta-analysis. EFORT Open Rev. 2021;6(1):35–49.
12. Raymond AC, McCann PA, Sarangi PP. Magnetic resonance scanning vs axillary radiography in the assessment of glenoid version for osteoarthritis. J Shoulder Elb Surg. 2013;22(8):1078–83.
13. Sabesan V, Callanan M, Ho J, Iannotti JP. Clinical and radiographic outcomes of total shoulder arthroplasty with bone graft for osteoarthritis with severe glenoid bone loss. J Bone Joint Surg Am. 2013;95(14):1290–6.
14. Nyffeler RW, Jost B, Pfirrmann CW, Gerber C. Measurement of glenoid version: conventional radiographs versus computed tomography scans. J Shoulder Elb Surg. 2003;12(5):493–6.
15. Friedman RJ, Hawthorne KB, Genez BM. The use of computerized tomography in the measurement of glenoid version. J Bone Joint Surg Am. 1992;74(7):1032–7.
16. Neyton L, Walch G, Nové-Josserand L, Edwards TB. Glenoid corticocancellous bone grafting after glenoid component removal in the treatment of glenoid loosening. J Shoulder Elb Surg. 2006;15(2):173–9.
17. Keller J, Bak S, Bigliani LU, Levine WN. Glenoid replacement in total shoulder arthroplasty. Orthopedics. 2006;29(3):221–6.

18. Amini MH, Ricchetti ET, Iannotti JP. Three-dimensional templating and use of standard instrumentation in primary anatomic total shoulder arthroplasty. JBJS Essent Surg Tech. 2017;7(3):e28.
19. Gauci MO, Cavalier M, Gonzalez JF, Holzer N, Baring T, Walch G, et al. Revision of failed shoulder arthroplasty: epidemiology, etiology, and surgical options. J Shoulder Elb Surg. 2020;29(3):541–9.
20. Shukla DR, McLaughlin RJ, Lee J, Nguyen NTV, Sanchez-Sotelo J. Automated three-dimensional measurements of version, inclination, and subluxation. Shoulder Elbow. 2020;12(1):31–7.
21. Freehill MT, Weick JW, Ponce BA, Bedi A, Haas D, Ruffino B, et al. Anatomic total shoulder arthroplasty: component size prediction with 3-dimensional preoperative digital planning. J Shoulder Elb Arthroplast. 2022;6:24715492221098818.

Preoperative Planning in Anatomic Shoulder Arthroplasty

3

A. De Vita, R. Russo, and F. Familiari

3.1 Introduction

The utilisation of total shoulder arthroplasty continues to grow. Proper implant positioning, particularly of the glenoid in anatomic total shoulder arthroplasty (ATSA), is paramount to achieving a good result and avoiding devastating complications and early failure. Preoperative planning software based on three-dimensional CT (3D CT) has revolutionized the surgeon's ability to visualize glenoid deformity and bone stock, plan corrective procedures for abnormal version, and visualize component position. Understanding the normal and degenerative shoulder anatomy is necessary for correct planning of anatomic total shoulder arthroplasty. The goal of anatomic total shoulder arthroplasty is to restore the premorbid state by recreating normal shoulder kinematics. This simple objective can, however, be challenging to achieve, as anatomy is subject to premorbid variations, in addition to distortions secondary to degenerative or traumatic changes [1]. Failure to restore anatomy and, therefore, provide a stable fulcrum will result in early implant failure secondary to glenoid loosening.

3.2 Anatomy

3.2.1 Humerus

Anatomy is critical to reproduce the patient's physiologic joint kinematics successfully. By virtue of its mobility, the glenohumeral joint is predisposed to instability.

A. De Vita · R. Russo · F. Familiari (✉)
Department of Orthopaedic and Trauma Surgery, Magna Graecia University, Catanzaro, Italy

Research Center on Musculoskeletal Health, Magna Graecia University, Catanzaro, Italy
e-mail: filippofamiliari@unicz.it

G. M. Marcheggiani Muccioli et al. (eds.), *Easy Planning in Elective Primary Orthopedic Procedures*, https://doi.org/10.1007/978-3-031-77006-7_3

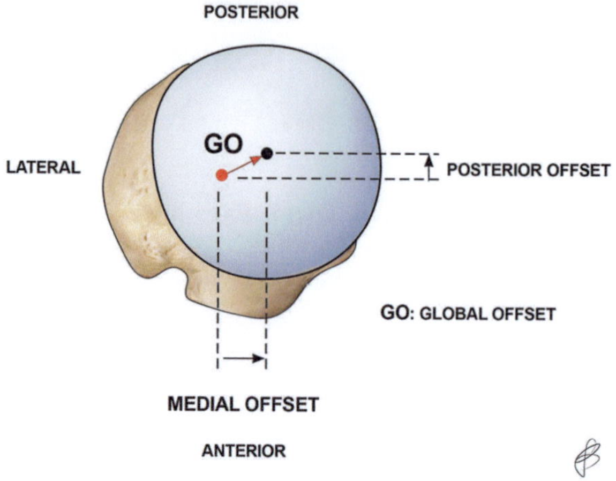

Fig. 3.1 Global Offset between the humeral canal and the center of the humeral head (medial and posterior).

One factor affecting stability is the radius of curvature mismatch between the humeral head and glenoid. Further, only 20–30% of the humeral head is in contact with the glenoid. The non-arthritic humeral head has a mean three-dimensional measured diameter of 46.2 ± 5.4 mm (range: 37.1–56.9 mm) and a humeral height of approximately 19 mm [2, 3]. The osteoarthritic head is flattened and widened with a mean diameter of 59 ± 9 mm [4]. The humeral head has the particularity to be elliptic in the periphery and become spherical in its central part, meaning that the cut surface will be about 2 mm larger from medial to lateral than from anterior to posterior [3]. The ratio between humeral head size and height is relatively constant [5]. Lastly, relative to the humeral canal, the head has a posterior and medial offset of 0.35–2.6 mm and 5.6–9.7 mm, respectively (Fig. 3.1) [1–6]. The mean neck-shaft angle (NSA) or inclination of the proximal humerus is approximately 135° but varies between 115° and 148°. Humeral head torsion is important in ATSA as it directly affects the joint center of rotation (COR) and thereby influences mobility in external rotation and shoulder stability [7, 8]. A cadaveric study by Pearl and Volk reported a mean humeral retroversion of 29.8° with a 95% confidence interval of 7°–52° (Fig. 3.2) [9]. While they used the trochlear axis as a reference, other reported values were based on the trans-epicondylar axis (which differs from 3° to 8°). Furthermore, current systems use a jig aligned on the forearm as a reference; in this case, a 10°–15° carrying angle must be added to the reported values (Fig. 3.2). Finally, the intramedullary canal not only becomes narrower but also increasingly retroverted from proximal to distal [10].

3.3 Glenoid

The glenoid seems relatively small and shallow compared to the humerus, with only 9 cm^2 of articular surface [11]. The glenoid is pear-shaped with a superior to an inferior dimension of 39 mm and an inferior glenoid width averaging 29 mm [3].

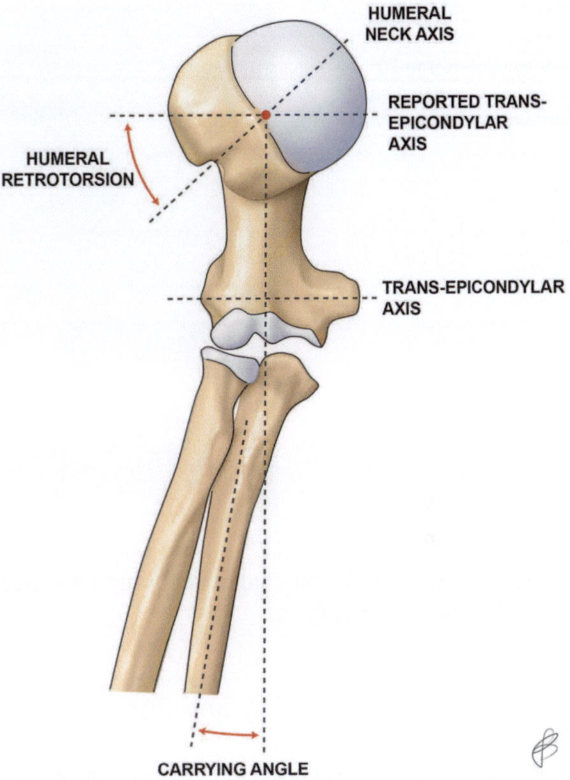

Fig. 3.2 Humeral head retroversion: using trans-epicondylar axis as reference, the retroversion is about 29.8°. In case using the forearm alignment, it is necessary to added 10°–15°.

There is a radii mismatch between the glenoid and humeral head, while the radius of curvature is greater in the anteroposterior than the superoinferior direction (41 mm vs. 32 mm) [12]. Biomechanically, perfect conformity leads to a more stable joint but increased stress on the glenoid. Reported three-dimensional CT-derived measures report mean normal glenoid retroversion of 6 ± 4° and inclination of 7 ± 5°. Retroversion has been correlated ($r = 0.7$, $P < 0.001$) to posterior humeral head subluxation (59% ± 7%) [13]. The contralateral shoulder may be a reliable model; side-to-side differences are limited to 5° in 95% of cases [14]. It is also important to assess the version in three dimensions, as in cases with >10° version, it is not solely direct posteriorly but also in superior, inferior, and anterior directions [15]. A further important indicator when performing ATSA is that the version of the inferior part of the glenoid shows substantially less variability compared to the upper part and should, therefore, be used as the preferred intraoperative landmark in order to achieve adequate implant positioning [16]. Concerning inclination, Moor et al. proposed the critical shoulder angle (CSA) as a measure of scapular morphology with the benefit of combining measurements of glenoid inclination and lateral acromion coverage [17]. They identified an angle inferior to 30° as being associated with primary shoulder osteoarthritis (Fig. 3.3). This finding is supported by

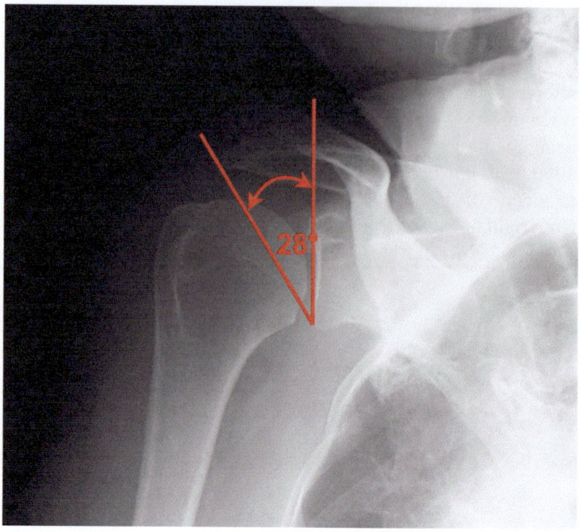

Fig. 3.3 Critical shoulder angle (CSA). In case of the angle is inferior to 30° could be associated with primary shoulder arthritis

subsequent biomechanical studies reporting increased joint reaction forces in the case of a lower CSA [18, 19].

3.4 Shoulder Stability and Rotator Cuff Functions

The rotator cuff and the horizontal force couple are critical for glenohumeral stability in the mid-range of motion [20]. At maximal degrees of motion, the ligament's function is crucial in granting joint stability. Both ligaments and muscles are essential to joint equilibrium after ATSA. Soft tissue balancing is evaluated between the subscapularis tendon and the posterior capsule, and it needs to be obtained in order to reach Matsen's criteria (40° of external rotation, 60° of internal rotation, and a 50% posterior shift of the humeral head over the glenoid) after ATSA [21].

3.5 Importance of Glenoid in Anatomic Total Shoulder Arthroplasty

Implantation of both glenoid and humeral components in ATSA is important for correct kinematics of the shoulder joint, but correct implantation of the glenoid component is a challenging yet critical aspect of the procedure. Glenoid component position is crucial for postoperative functional outcomes and implant longevity in TSA [22]. Improper glenoid component positioning is a significant risk factor for early glenoid failure, the most common mode of failure in TSA [23, 24]. Malposition of the glenoid component creates an articulation that fails to restore normal joint biomechanics and can impart significantly greater stress at the bone–implant interface, causing implant micromotion and subsequent loosening and failure [25–27].

Ultimately, this leads to inferior clinical outcomes [28]. Inferiorly inclined glenoid components are associated with an increased incidence of radiolucent lines on post-operative radiographs, and increased glenoid retroversion and non-neutral rotation are associated with decreased range of motion, humeral head subluxation or dislocation, and loosening [28, 29]. If glenoid retroversion cannot be completely corrected without severely compromising glenoid bone stock, the glenoid component may be placed in excessive retroversion. Iannotti et al. showed that retroversion greater than 20° can lead to center peg perforation of the anterior glenoid wall [29].

A clear understanding of the patient's anatomy is crucial to implementing patient-specific strategies to properly place the glenoid component and avoid complications associated with improper component positioning. For this reason, it is essential to execute preoperative planning.

3.6 Preoperative Evaluation

The first steps in planning for ATSA include obtaining patient history, performing a thorough physical examination, and obtaining basic radiographs. Cuff evaluation tests like the Jobe test, Lift-off test, Bear hug test, and Patte test are mandatory to assess the validity of cuff function. The routine shoulder radiograph series includes anteroposterior (AP), Grashey, scapular "Y," and axillary views. The Grashey view (real A-P view) demonstrates glenohumeral joint space narrowing (Fig. 3.4), and the axillary view allows for visualization of the glenoid, including version abnormalities and various anterior or posterior wear patterns, which may influence implant placement and augmentation strategies. Additionally, MRI is crucial to

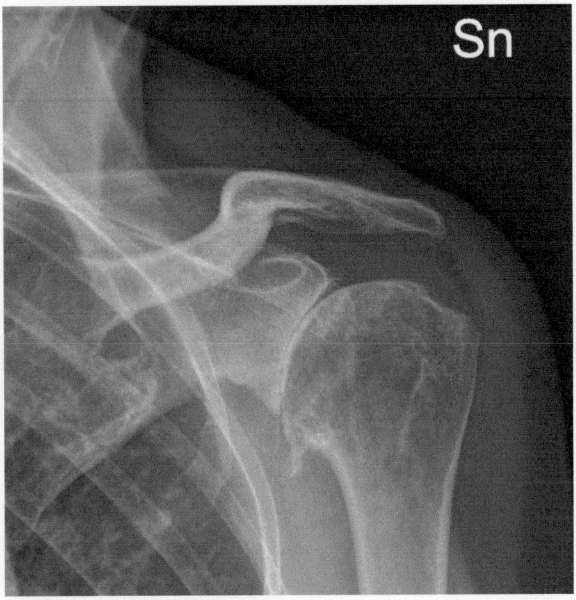

Fig. 3.4 The Grashey view (real A-P view) demonstrates glenohumeral joint space narrowing

understand the conditions of the rotator cuff tendons and muscles. The integrity of the rotator cuff tendons and muscles is mandatory to perform ATSA. 2D and 3D CT scans provide additional detail and improved accuracy to evaluate glenohumeral deformity. The use of CT has become much more common for the preoperative assessment of an arthritic shoulder as the use of templating software has evolved. It is important to ensure the appropriate orientation of the CT cuts during formatting to be perpendicular to the axis of the scapula. For optimal evaluation and planning for reconstruction, it is also recommended that the imaging cuts be oriented perpendicular to the surface of the glenoid. The scapula is 20°–30° anteverted in relation to the coronal plane, and this must be accounted for as every 1° of scapular abduction in the coronal plane results in a 0.42° increase in measured glenoid anteversion [30]. After imaging has been obtained, the glenoid is analyzed in a variety of ways to assess the glenoid version, bone loss, and humeral head subluxation. The Friedman angle is commonly used to assess the glenoid version and is calculated using axial scapula imaging. A line is drawn from the scapula's medial tip through the glenoid fossa's midpoint (Friedman line). A second line perpendicular to this is determined to be neutral, and the angle between the second line and a third line connecting the anterior and posterior rims of the glenoid is the calculated version (Fig. 3.5) [31]. The global glenoid inclination or β-angle may be used to determine vertical glenoid inclination in ATSA. This angle is calculated on AP or coronal imaging by the intersection of a line parallel to the floor of the supraspinatus fossa and a second line parallel to the glenoid face [32]. Daggett et al. found that β-angle is most accurately reproduced on either 3D CT scans or 2D CT imaging reformatted in the scapular plane, whereas plain radiographs and unformatted 2D CTs are unreliable methods of measurement [33]. A combination of meticulous assessment of tests for rotator cuff function and imaging is useful to confirm surgical strategy.

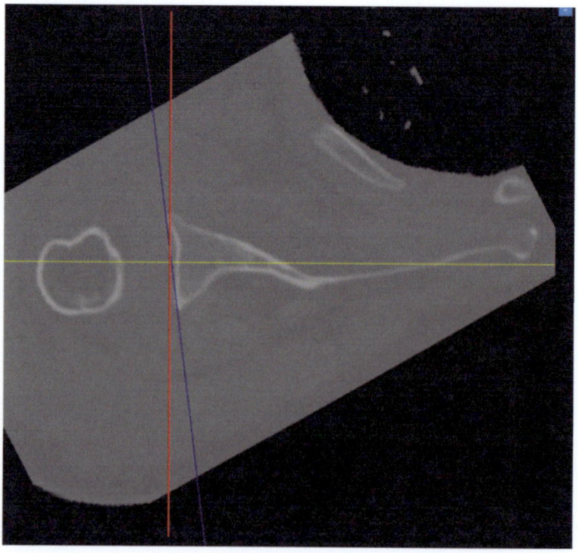

Fig. 3.5 To calculate the retroversion of the glenoid, it is important to drawn a Freedman line (yellow). Angle between the blue and red line indicate glenoid retroversion

3.7 Humeral Head Size and Position

Restoring the humeral head anatomy and center of rotation (COR) is necessary to avoid implant loosening and restore range of motion. Deviations from the anatomic COR most often result in a medialized center of rotation or overstuffing of the humeral implant, resulting in altered glenohumeral mechanics [34]. Such overstuffing can lead to increased stress on the rotator cuff and result in early failure. Studies have shown that as few as 2.5 mm of superior translation of the humeral head may lead to impingement [35]. The humeral head height, neck-shaft angle, and radius of curvature are often used to determine the premorbid anatomy; however, this is often a challenge in an arthritic humeral head. In addition to proper sizing of the humeral head, the appreciation of its position relative to the glenoid is also important. Proper restoration of the humeral head can help balance soft tissues that mantain this relationship, but the morphology of the glenoid also lplays a significant role. Two common methods are used to measure the amount of humeral head subluxation on a CT scan. The scapula axis method measures the anteroposterior length of the humeral head located posterior to the scapular axis (Friedman line) compared with the anteroposterior diameter of the humeral head (Fig. 3.6). The mediatrice method uses a similar calculation; however, the reference line is perpendicular to the middle of the glenoid joint surface. This method is considered more of a glenohumeral axis rather than the scapulohumeral assessment of the Friedman line. A ratio greater than 55% is defined as posterior subluxation.

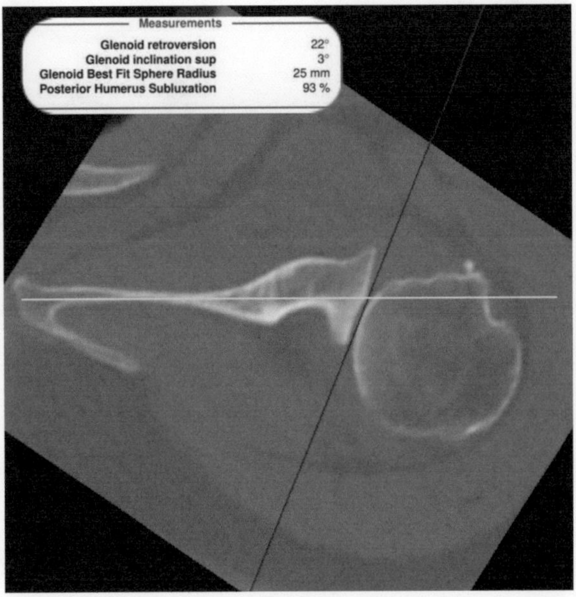

Fig. 3.6 Humeral head posterior subluxation: the scapula axis method measures the anteroposterior length of the humeral head located posterior to the scapular axis (Friedman line—yellow) compared with the anteroposterior diameter of the humeral head (in this case 93% posterior subluxation)

3.8 Glenoid Version

Different methods have been described to measure version based on CT imaging. The technique described by Friedman et al. [31] uses the scapular axis, drawn from the midpoint of the glenoid fossa to the root of the scapular spine on an axial cut. This axis is typically chosen on the axial image of the glenoid, just inferior to the coracoid process. A line drawn perpendicular to the scapular axis is considered the neutral version. The angle formed between the line or neutral version and a line between the anterior and posterior margins of the glenoid represents the version. More posterior wear of the glenoid results in retroversion, which is represented in negative degrees (Fig. 3.6). The most used assessment of glenoid morphology is the Walch classification (Fig. 3.7), which was initially described in 1999 using 2D CT imaging [36]. Walch originally described three main morphologic types: type A, in which the humeral head was centered; type B, in which the humeral head was subluxated posteriorly; and type C, characterized by a glenoid retroversion of at least 25°. Type A was further subclassified into A1 or A2 for minor or major central glenoid erosion, respectively. Type B glenoids were subdivided into types B1 and B2, with B2 glenoids demonstrating a biconcave morphology. In 2016, Bercik et al [37]. modify the Walch classification with the description of the B3 and D glenoids. B3 glenoids are characterized by posterior wear and a mono-concave articular

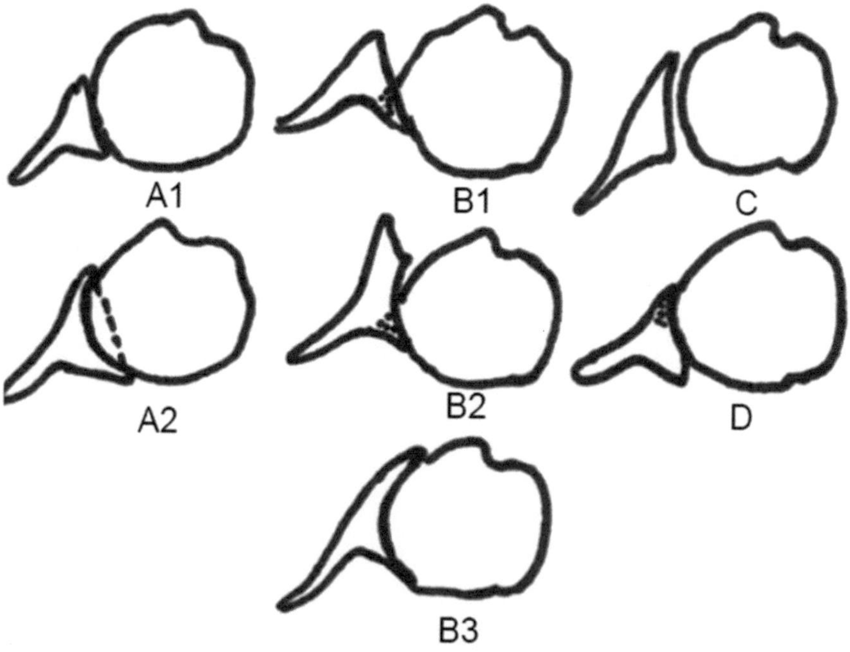

Fig. 3.7 The modified Walch classification of the glenoid. Reproduced with permission by Elsevier from Walch et al. [36]

surface, with at least 15° of retroversion or 70% posterior humeral head subluxation. Type D glenoids are characterized by any level of glenoid anteversion [37]. In addition, the authors further categorized type C glenoids that are dysplastic glenoids (Fig. 3.7).

3.9 Preoperative Anatomical Total Shoulder Arthroplasty Templating

In our practice, we start to plan an ATSA with a CT evaluation. A 2D CT scan can be used to determine the glenoid version and humeral head morphology, as previously described in the first step. Based on anatomic landmarks, we estimate the pin placement needed before reaming to obtain the required correction. Optimal glenoid implant position can be achieved in cases of minimal deformity (inferior of 10° of retroversion). Preoperative glenoid retroversion greater than 10° prevents placement of the glenoid implant within 10° of the ideal retroversion [38]. However, when comparing preoperative planning done on 2D imaging, reevaluation with 3D reconstruction resulted in a change of implant selection in 14% of cases and a change from planned TSA to reverse TSA in 8% of cases [39]. For this reason, we always prefer to use 3D templating software for planning ATSA. Templating with 3D reconstructions of imaging allows for virtual implantation, which facilitates visualization of selected implants and results in more reliable prediction of implants. Preoperative planning using 3D reconstruction of a 2D CT scan can match the selected glenoid size, head size, and head thickness 100% of the time when compared with those selected preoperatively [40]. The evolution of modern templating software has exploded in recent years, with multiple implant designers offering their own software programs to allow for virtual preoperative planning using patient imaging studies. A standard thin slice (<1 mm) 2D CT scan of the shoulder with all the scapula included is obtained by a patient and is reformatted by these various software programs with 3D reconstruction of the scapula and the humerus to help identify accurate landmarks and assess version, inclination of the glenoid, and subluxation of humeral head (Fig. 3.8). In addition, these programs allow for virtual implantation of glenoid and humeral implants into the 3D bone reconstructions. Surgeons can assess guide pin placement into the glenoid (Fig. 3.8), whether there is center peg perforation risk, and even determine the need for augmented implants in cases of significant posterior glenoid wear (Fig. 3.9). In our practice, we prefer to use a commercially available 3D planning tool: BLUEPRINT, Wright Medical, Memphis, TN. It is important to have a good evaluation of shoulder deformity not only with software for planning ATSA but also with 2D CT to analyze the images independently and appreciate bony anatomy free of any software influence. This is because the software programs tended to show increased measures of superior inclination, retroversion of the glenoid, and posterior subluxation of the humeral head. Some papers demonstrated higher reliability of measurements obtained by surgeons [41]. To obtain good implantation of ATSA, we think it is important to respect the five rules described by Giles Walch: (1) less than 10° of glenoid implant

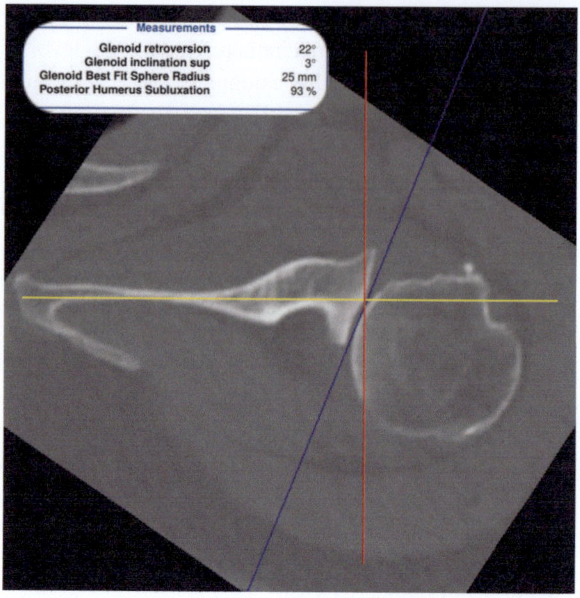

Fig. 3.8 B2 glenoid. The angle between the red and blue line indicates the glenoid retroversion (in this case 22° of retroversion)

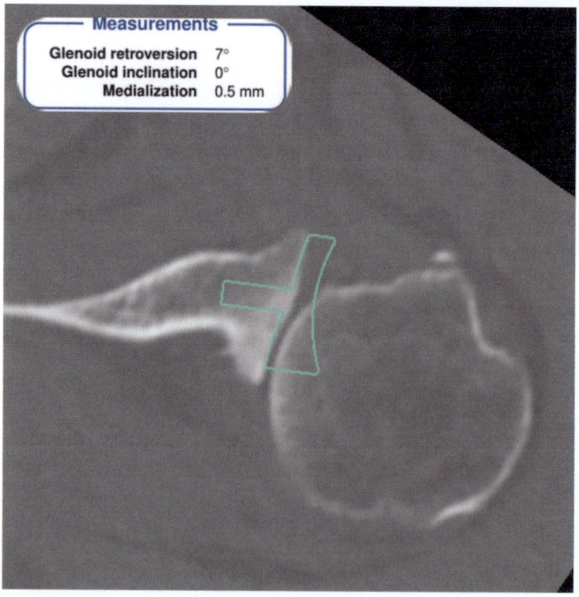

Fig. 3.9 B2 glenoid. Augmented posterior implant to correct significant posterior glenoid wear maintaining 7° of retroversion

retroversion; (2) less than 10° of glenoid implant superior inclination; (3) 80% of the glenoid implant seating; (4) less than 80% of humeral head subluxation; (5) subchondral bone preservation. These rules help to avoid premature implant failure for loosening of the components, avoid implant instability, and help to preserve as much bone stock as possible in case of revision surgery.

Take Home Messages

1. A clear understanding of the patient's anatomy is crucial to avoid complications associated with improper component positioning.
2. Preoperative MRI is crucial to assess the integrity of the rotator cuff tendons and muscles to perform ATSA.
3. CT is mandatory for the use of templating software.
4. Templating with 3D imaging reconstructions allows for virtual implantation, which facilitates visualization of selected implants and results in more reliable prediction of implants.
5. Respect the five rules described by Giles Walch: (1) less than 10° of glenoid implant retroversion; (2) less than 10° of glenoid implant superior inclination; (3) 80% of the glenoid implant seating; (4) less than 80% of humeral head subluxation; (5) subchondral bone preservation.
6. The use of these technologies must be recognized as supplements to conducting ATSA and not as a substitute for the intraoperative decision-making of the surgeon because many dynamic aspects of the functioning shoulder cannot be adequately measured with static imaging.

References

1. Getz CL, Ricchetti ET, Verborgt O, Brolin TJ. Normal and pathoanatomy of the arthritic shoulder: considerations for shoulder arthroplasty. J Am Acad Orthop Surg. 2019;27:e1068–76.
2. Boileau P, Walch G. The three-dimensional geometry of the proximal humerus. Implications for surgical technique and prosthetic design. J Bone Joint Surg (Br). 1997;79-B:857–65.
3. Iannotti JP, Gabriel JP, Schneck SL, Evans BG, Misra S. The normal glenohumeral relationships: an anatomical study of one hundred and forty shoulders. J Bone Joint Surg Am. 1992;74-A:491–500.
4. Knowles NK, Carroll MJ, Keener JD, Ferreira LM, Athwal GS. A comparison of normal and osteoarthritic humeral head size and morphology. J Shoulder Elb Surg. 2016;25:502–9.
5. Hertel R, Knothe U, Ballmer FT. Geometry of the proximal humerus and implications for prosthetic design. J Shoulder Elb Surg. 2002;11:331–8.
6. Barth J, Garret J, Boutsiadis A, et al. Is global humeral head offset related to intramedullary canal width? A computer tomography morphometric study. J Exp Orthop. 2018;5:35.
7. Bryce C, Davison AC, Okita N, Lewis GS, Sharkey NA, Armstrong AD. A biomechanical study of posterior glenoid bone loss and humeral head translation. J Shoulder Elb Surg. 2010;19:994–1002.
8. Ovesen J, Nielsen S. Prosthesis position in shoulder arthroplasty: a cadaver study of the humeral component. Acta Orthop Scand. 1985;56:330–1.
9. Pearl ML, Volk AG. Retroversion of the proximal humerus in relationship to prosthetic replacement arthroplasty. J Shoulder Elb Surg. 1995;4:286–9.
10. Robertson DD, Yuan J, Bigliani LU, El F, Yamaguchi K. Three-dimensional analysis of the proximal part of the humerus: relevance to arthroplasty. J Bone Joint Surg Am. 2000;82-A:1594–602.
11. Kwon YW, Powell KA, Yum JK, Brems JJ, Iannotti JP. Use of three-dimensional computed tomography for the analysis of the glenoid anatomy. J Shoulder Elb Surg. 2005;14:85–90.
12. McPherson EJ, Friedman RJ, An YH, Chokesi R, Dooley RL. Anthropometric study of normal glenohumeral relationships. J Shoulder Elb Surg. 1997;6:105–12.

13. Gauci MO, Deransart P, Chaoui J, et al. Three-dimensional geometry of the normal shoulder: a software analysis. J Shoulder Elb Surg. 2020;29:e468–77.
14. Verhaegen F, Plessers K, Verborgt O, Scheys L, De Beer P. Can the contralateral scapula be used as a reliable template to reconstruct the eroded scapula during shoulder arthroplasty? J Shoulder Elb Surg. 2018;27:1133–8.
15. Sharkey NA, Marder RA. The rotator cuff opposes superior translation of the humeral head. Am J Sports Med. 1995;23:270–5.
16. De Wilde LF, Verstraeten T, Speeckaert W, Karelse A. Reliability of the glenoid plane. J Shoulder Elb Surg. 2010;19:414–22.
17. Moor BK, Bouaicha S, Rothenfluh DA, Sukthankar A, Gerber C. Is there an association between the individual anatomy of the scapula and the development of rotator cuff tears or osteoarthritis of the glenohumeral joint? A radiological study of the critical shoulder angle. J Bone Joint Surg (Br). 2013;95-B:935–41.
18. Engelhardt C, Farron A, Becce F, Place N, Pioletti DP, Terrier A. Effects of glenoid inclination and acromion index on humeral head translation and glenoid articular cartilage strain. J Shoulder Elb Surg. 2017;26:157–64.
19. Viehöfer AF, Snedeker JG, Baumgartner D, Gerber C. Glenohumeral joint reaction forces increase with critical shoulder angles representative of osteoarthritis: a biomechanical analysis. J Orthop Res. 2016;34:1047–52.
20. Goetti P, Denard PJ, Collin P, Ibrahim M, Hoffmeyer P, Lädermann A. Shoulder biomechanics in normal and selected pathological conditions. EFORT Open Rev. 2020;5:508–18.
21. Bergmann G, Graichen F, Bender A, et al. In vivo gleno-humeral joint loads during forward flexion and abduction. J Biomech. 2011;44:1543–52.
22. Burns DM, Frank T, Whyne CM, Henry PD. Glenoid component positioning and guidance techniques in anatomic and reverse total shoulder arthroplasty: a systematic review and meta-analysis. Shoulder Elbow. 2019;11:16e28.
23. Horneff JGI, Serra Lopez VM. Preoperative planning for anatomic total shoulder arthroplasty. J Am Acad Orthop Surg. 2022;30:e1207e16.
24. Matsen FA 3rd, Clinton J, Lynch J, Bertelsen A, Richardson ML. Glenoid component failure in total shoulder arthroplasty. J Bone Joint Surg Am. 2008;90:885e96.
25. Farron A, Terrier A, Buchler P. Risks of loosening of a prosthetic glenoid implanted in retroversion. J Shoulder Elb Surg. 2006;15:521e6.
26. Iannotti JP, Norris TR. Influence of preoperative factors on outcome of shoulder arthroplasty for glenohumeral osteoarthritis. J Bone Joint Surg Am. 2003;85:251e8.
27. Sears BW, Johnston PS, Ramsey ML, Williams GR. Glenoid bone loss in primary total shoulder arthroplasty: evaluation and management. J Am Acad Orthop Surg. 2012;20:604e13.
28. Gregory TM, Sankey A, Augereau B, Vandenbussche E, Amis A, Emery R, et al. Accuracy of glenoid component placement in total shoulder arthroplasty and its effect on clinical and radiological outcome in a retrospective, longitudinal, monocentric open study. PLoS One. 2013;8:e75791.
29. Iannotti JP, Greeson C, Downing D, Sabesan V, Bryan JA. Effect of glenoid deformity on glenoid component placement in primary shoulder arthroplasty. J Shoulder Elb Surg. 2012;21:48e55.
30. Bryce CD, Davison AC, Lewis GS, Wang L, Flemming DJ, Armstrong AD. Two-dimensional glenoid version measurements vary with coronal and sagittal scapular rotation. J Bone Joint Surg Am. 2010;92:692e9.
31. Friedman RJ, Hawthorne KB, Genez BM. The use of computerized tomography in the measurement of glenoid version. J Bone Joint Surg Am. 1992;74:1032–7.
32. Maurer A, Fucentese SF, Pfirrmann CW, Wirth SH, Djahangiri A, Jost B, et al. Assessment of glenoid inclination on routine clinical radiographs and computed tomography examinations of the shoulder. J Shoulder Elb Surg. 2012;21:1096e103.
33. Daggett M, Werner B, Gauci MO, Chaoui J, Walch G. Comparison of glenoid inclination angle using different clinical imaging modalities. J Shoulder Elb Surg. 2016;25:180e5.

34. Buzzell JE, Lutton DM, Shyr Y, Neviaser RJ, Lee DH. Reliability and accuracy of templating the proximal humeral component for shoulder arthroplasty. J Shoulder Elb Surg. 2009;18:728–33.
35. Favre P, Moor B, Snedeker JG, Gerber C. Influence of component positioning on impingement in conventional total shoulder arthroplasty. Clin Biomech. 2008;23:175–83.
36. Walch G, Badet R, Boulahia A, Khoury A. Morphologic study of the glenoid in primary glenohumeral osteoarthritis. J Arthroplast. 1999;14:756–60.
37. Bercik MJ, Kruse K, Yalizis M, Gauci MO, Chaoui J, Walch G. A modification to the Walch classification of the glenoid in primary glenohumeral osteoarthritis using three-dimensional imaging. J Shoulder Elbow Surg. 2016;25:1601–6.
38. Hendel MD, Bran JA, Barsoum WK, et al. Comparison of patient-specific instruments with standard surgical instruments in determining glenoid component position: a randomized prospective clinical trial. J Bone Joint Surg Am. 2012;94:2167–75.
39. Werner BS, Hudek R, Burkhart KJ, Gohlke F. The influence of three dimensional planning on decision-making in total shoulder arthroplasty. J Shoulder Elb Surg. 2017;26:1477–83.
40. Cho SH, Jeong J. Radiologic results of three-dimensional templating for total shoulder arthroplasty. Clin Orthop Surg. 2020;12:232–7.
41. Erickson BJ, Chalmers PN, Denard P, et al. Does commercially available shoulder arthroplasty preoperative planning software agree with surgeon measurements of version, inclination, and subluxation? Shoulder Elbow Surg. 2021;30:413–20.

RTSA for Primary Osteoarthritis: Preoperative Planning

4

M. Monetta, M. Riva, F. Tortorella, F. Coliva, M. Cavallo, and E. Guerra

4.1 Introduction and Biomechanics

Reverse total shoulder arthroplasty (RTSA) has become a common surgical procedure for both elective surgery and for fracture treatment. The first reverse implant was designed by Charles Neer II in 1972 but Paul Grammont's Trompette is considered to be the first "modern" design.

RTSA is an orthopedic device that is meant to modify the normal biomechanics of the shoulder and it is meant to work without the rotator cuff tendons and muscles action. The usual concavity and convexity of the shoulder joint are inverted: the humeral head is replaced by a concavity placed on the humeral prosthesis and the glenoid surface is replaced by a spherical device that is the glenosphere. This simple, but still brilliant, modification changes significantly the position of the center of rotation of the joint medializing and lowering it (Fig. 4.1). In this way the deltoid muscle fibers are tensioned and positioned in a condition that allows them to generate an abduction movement from the very first degrees, even without the supporting action of the rotator cuff muscles, particularly of the supraspinatus.

4.2 Classifications of Glenoid Bone Defects

Several well-established classification systems are available to describe glenoid deformity in the primary setting of osteoarthritis. In 1999, Gilles Walch proposed a prognostic classification of glenoid morphology using computed tomography scans to measure glenoid retroversion and different erosion patterns. These findings still have important implications for prosthetic replacement of the shoulder nowadays.

M. Monetta · M. Riva · F. Tortorella · F. Coliva · M. Cavallo · E. Guerra (✉)
Shoulder and Elbow Unit – IRCCS, Istituto Ortopedico Rizzoli, Bologna, Italy
e-mail: enrico.guerra@ior.it

G. M. Marcheggiani Muccioli et al. (eds.), *Easy Planning in Elective Primary Orthopedic Procedures*, https://doi.org/10.1007/978-3-031-77006-7_4

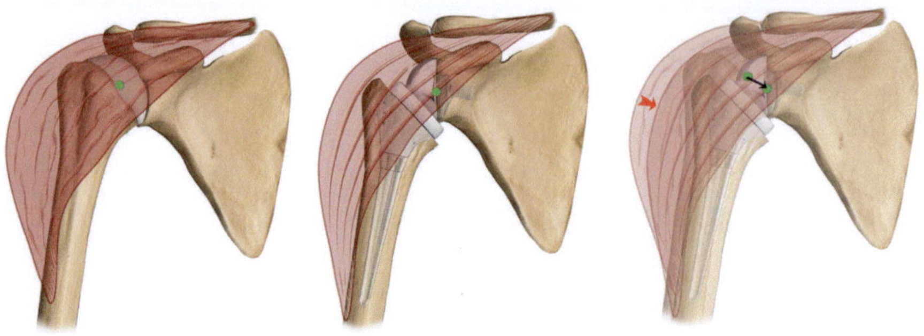

Fig. 4.1 Biomechanical changes of RTSA. The center of rotation is medialized and lowered and the deltoid fibers are already tensioned in adduction.

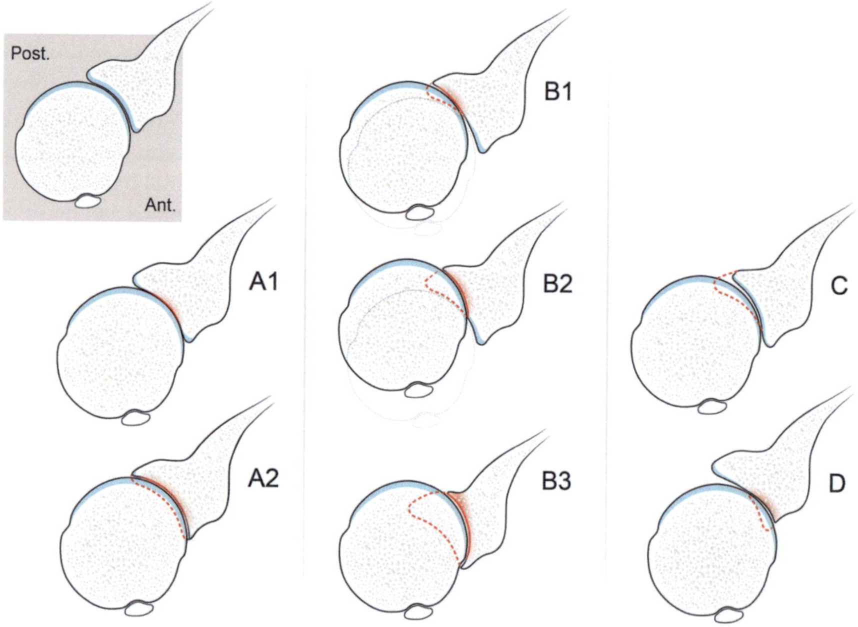

Fig. 4.2 Walch classification of glenoid morphology.

According to the original Walch classification [1] (Fig. 4.2), there are three types of glenoid morphology:

- Type A (59%): centered humeral head and minor (A1, 43%) or major (A2, 16%) central and symmetric erosion of the glenoid with a mean glenoid retroversion of 11.5°. In order to distinguish between A1 and A2 glenoid, a line passing between anterior and posterior margins of the glenoid is drawn: if the medial aspect of the humeral head crosses this line, the glenoid is considered type A2 [2, 3].

- Type B (32%): humeral head subluxated posteriorly and asymmetric load distribution with various degrees of posterior glenoid wear. In the two subgroups that were identified, the B1 glenoid (17%) refers to a posterior subluxation without glenoid erosion, while in the B2 (15%) a posterior wear occurs, and the glenoid is characterized by a biconcave aspect. According to Walch's studies, the posterior wear happens as a consequence of static posterior subluxation of the humeral head with secondary erosion of the posterior aspect of the glenoid. In the B group, the mean glenoid retroversion was found to be around 18°; however, in type B2 glenoids, posterior wear may significantly increase glenoid retroversion.
- Type C (9%) glenoids are defined by a retroversion of more than 25°, regardless of the erosion patterns. The origin of the retroversion is predominantly dysplastic, with early development of osteoarthritis.

Later on, in 2016, Bercik et al. [2] proposed several modifications to the original classification, with the addition of two other subtypes of glenoid wear. Type B3 glenoid is defined as a monoconcave concentric glenoid with at least 15° of retroversion and at least 70% of subluxation of the humeral head posteriorly. The B2 glenoids may develop into a B3 as increased erosion destroys the paleoglenoid. On the other hand, type D glenoids are characterized by any level of anteversion with or without humeral head anterior subluxation.

The Favard classification (Fig. 4.3) [4] describes different patterns of glenoid erosion in the coronal plane in patients affected by cuff tear arthropathy (CTA):

- Type E0: CTA without glenoid erosion.
- Type E1: concentric glenoid erosion.
- Type E2: biconcave glenoid with superior erosion.
- Type E3: monoconcave glenoid with superior erosion.
- Type E4: Anteroinferior glenoid erosion with anteroinferior subluxation of the humeral head.

4.3 Assessment of Glenoid Morphology

A thorough preoperative assessment of glenoid morphology is essential during the surgical planning phase for the correct selection and positioning of the glenoid component. Radiographic assessment includes true (Grashey) anteroposterior view, axillary view, and scapular Y view. In order to study glenoid bone defects, computed tomography is the most accurate diagnostic modality. However, the standard CT-2D measurement techniques are subject to high variability due to the influence of the patient's positioning within the scanner [5]. Three reference points are commonly used to reorient the imaging planes (the "corrected" axial, coronal, and sagittal planes) to the anatomic plane of the scapula: (1) the junction of the scapular spine

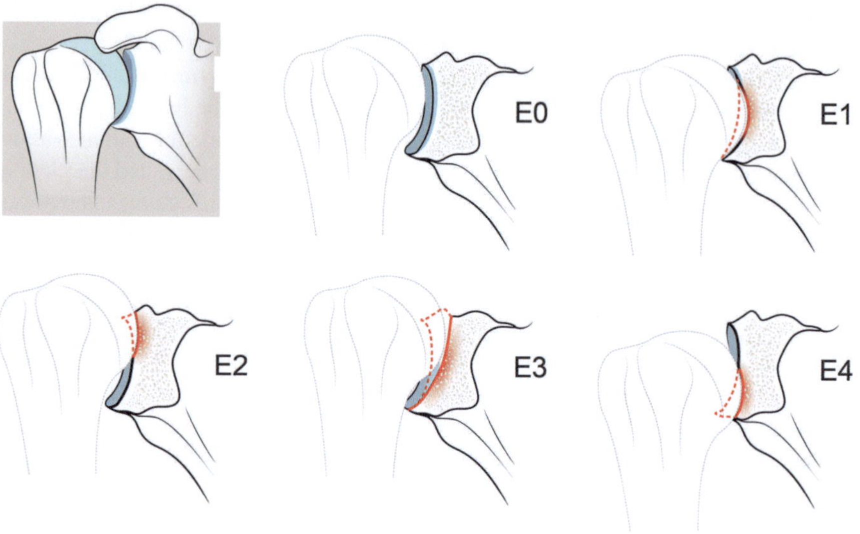

Fig. 4.3 Favard classification of glenoid morphology. Copyright of Maria Pia Cumani, 2024. All rights reserved

with the medial margin of the scapula, (2) the center of the glenoid, and (3) the inferior tip of the scapula. Over the last decade, three-dimensional (3D) measurements of glenoid morphology became increasingly used and acknowledged as an essential reference in preoperative planning, as they offer a more comprehensive volumetric method for the quantification of glenoid bone loss [3, 6, 7]. Modern software is available and provide a 3D reconstruction of the entire scapula, a graphic visualization of the bone defect, as well as precise measurements of glenoid version, inclination, and virtual positioning of the implants [8, 9]. Planning software builds a 3D model of patients' shoulders starting from segmented CT scan DICOM files allowing such measurements and predicting postoperative range of motion based on implant positioning and bony architecture.

As previously mentioned, glenoid version and inclination are essential parameters to be considered during reverse shoulder arthroplasty (RSA) planning, as they are subject to pathological changes due to the osteoarthritic process. The orientation of the glenoid is of paramount importance for joint biomechanics and accurate selection and positioning of the glenoid component. There are no standardized guidelines in the literature for optimal glenoid implant version, inclination, and lateralization in case of severe osteoarthritis and glenoid wear. In general, placing the glenoid component in a neutral version or in slight retroversion is suggested. Preoperative planning has become essential for characterizing a patient's specific glenoid bone loss [10, 11] and for the "correction" required during surgery. Normal glenoid version varies between 2° of anteversion and 9° of retroversion [12]. In most studies, is reported close to 0° or with slight retroversion and typically less than 10° [13]. However, it has a high grade of variability, whereas arthritic shoulders generally have higher grades of retroversion. Measurement of glenoid version is usually performed on a 2D CT axial section using the Friedman method. The Friedman line passes through the long axis of the scapula from the tip of the medial border to the center of the glenoid: neutral version of the glenoid happens when the line joining the anterior and posterior margin of the glenoid is perpendicular to the "Friedman Line." If the posterior margin of the glenoid is medial to the line of neutral version, then the glenoid is retroverted; on the other hand, if the anterior margin is medial to that line, the glenoid is anteverted. Furthermore, because of the spiral configuration of the glenoid, retroversion decreases in the superior to inferior direction, with an average value of 1° ± 3° in the middle section [14, 15]. The quantification of the glenoid version is described by the alfa-angle (α) (Fig. 4.4a) between the line of neutral version and the line across the anterior and posterior glenoid margins, excluding osteophytes.

The erosive process compromises the orientation of the articular surface. One of the most common glenoid wear patterns is posterior erosion resulting in retroversion. Posterior glenoid bone loss can cause static posterior subluxation of the humeral head due to altered biomechanics and this condition can lead to inferior outcomes when a total shoulder arthroplasty is performed [16]. Posterior bone loss can be quantified by measuring the distance between the posterior glenoid and a line perpendicular to the Friedman line, passing through the anterior margin of the glenoid (Fig. 4.4b) [3]. There is a significant correlation between glenoid retroversion and posterior subluxation of the humeral head referring to the scapular plane [17]. The presence of glenohumeral osteophytes has to be considered during the planning phase, as they can alter angle measurements. This is particularly important for the correspondence between planning and intraoperative findings [10].

As mentioned above, another critical morphologic parameter that has to be assessed in preoperative planning is glenoid inclination. The intrinsic glenoid inclination is defined as the angle between the floor of the supraspinatus fossa and the glenoid fossa line, known as the *beta angle* (Fig. 4.5), as described by Maurer et al. [18]. As shown in a cadaveric study conducted by Churchill et al., the glenoid inclination has high variability, with a range from −7° to 15.8° in men and − 1.5° to 15.3° in women [19]. Traditional measurements of glenoid inclination, including the *beta* angle, and its complementary angle, called the TSA angle (Fig. 4.6),

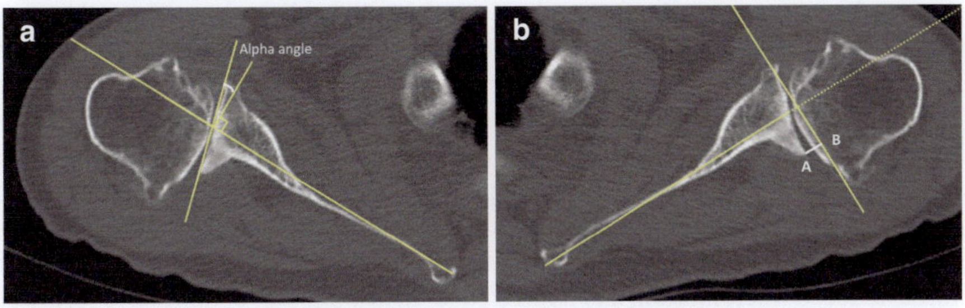

Fig. 4.4 (**a**) Alpha angle of glenoid version (**b**). Posterior glenoid loss (A–B)

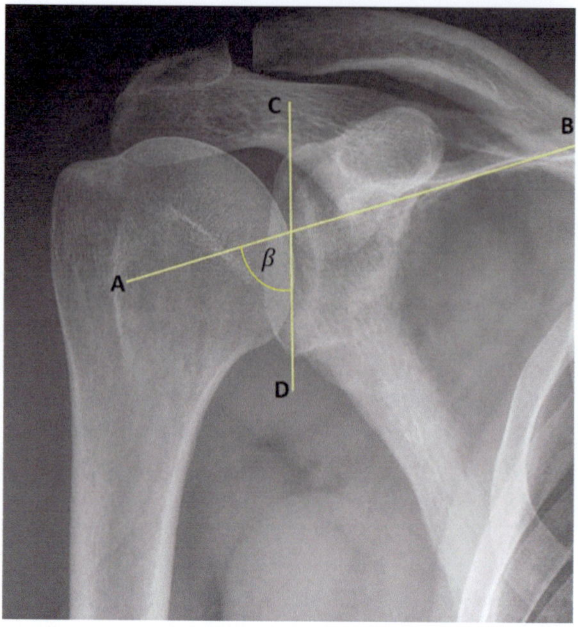

Fig. 4.5 The beta angle formed by the line passing through the floor of the supraspinatus fossa (A–B) and the glenoid fossa line (C–D)

consider the entire glenoid fossa, which is relevant when planning a total shoulder arthroplasty. Instead, when planning a reverse shoulder arthroplasty (RSA), the attention should be focused on measuring the inclination of the inferior half of the glenoid, where the baseplate is implanted, in order to avoid underestimation of the inclination with the measure provided by the beta angle. Boileau et al. introduced the "RSA angle" to provide a reliable measure of the inclination of the inferior aspect of the native glenoid, which is consistently superior to the inclination of the entire glenoid fossa. The RSA angle is defined as the angle between the line passing through the inferior part of the glenoid fossa, where the baseplate is implanted, and the line perpendicular to the floor of the supraspinatus fossa. The preoperative measure of the RSA angle allows to estimate the proper amount of correction necessary for achieving neutral inclination when positioning the baseplate [20].

Despite the well-established importance of glenoid orientation as a factor that significantly affects the outcomes of shoulder replacement, there is still no consensus on the optimal positioning and orientation of the baseplate. The debate on whether a neutral or inferior tilt is advisable is still ongoing; however, it is a widely held opinion the importance of avoiding superior inclination of the implant, which is associated with increased risk of aseptic loosening, scapular notching, and reduced ROM [21]. An inferior glenoid tilt of 10° was found to be associated with a reduced risk of dislocation when compared to a neutral tilt [22]. Furthermore, according to a biomechanical study conducted by Gutierrez et al. [23], positioning the glenoid with an inferior inclination leads to a decreased overall magnitude of force, reduced micromotion, and a more equal distribution of compressive forces at the baseplate level. However, a prospective randomized clinical study found no

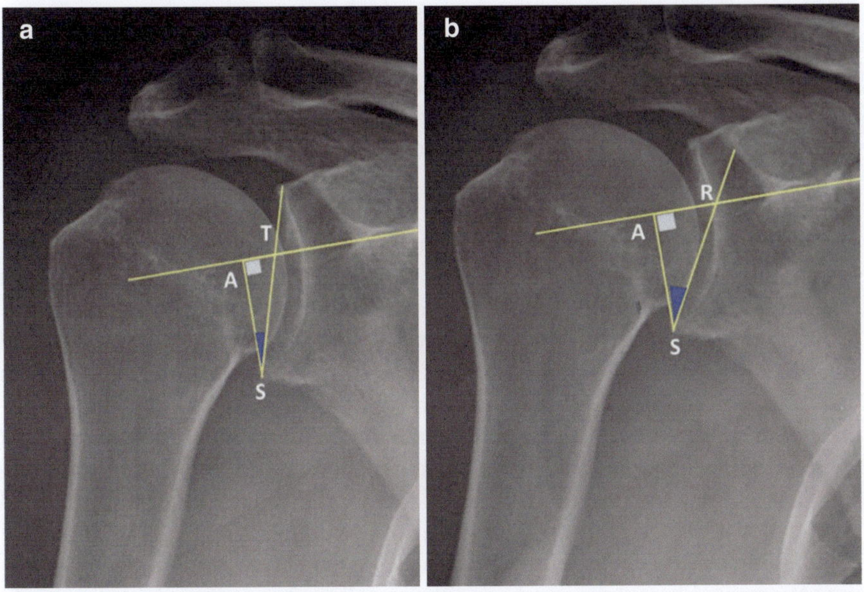

Fig. 4.6 (**a**) TSA angle: the complementary angle of the beta angle, formed by the glenoid fossa line and the perpendicular to the supraspinatus fossa line. (**b**) RSA angle: Point R (the intersection between the line passing through the supraspinatus fossa and the glenoid); Point S (inferior aspect of the glenoid); Point A (intersection between the supraspinatus fossa line and the perpendicular line originating from point S)

clinical or radiographic advantages in placing the baseplate with 10° inferior tilt compared to a neutral inclination [24].

To date, no agreement has been reached on a standardized approach to guide surgeons in the management of bone loss and the optimal point of baseplate placement remains an open debate. Placing the lower aspect of the glenosphere in alignment with the inferior glenoid rim was suggested to reduce scapular notching and lead to a better range of motion [25]. Several studies have tried to assess common patterns of distribution of bone loss to identify regions of adequate bone stock to support implant fixation and screw positioning in the largest available mass of bone [26] in order to plan potential screw trajectories before starting the surgery. Optimal screw placement was defined as the achievement of maximal screw length, and far cortical fixation and placement in one of the three scapular pillars : the coracoid pillar (the aiming point for the superior screw), the scapular spine pillar (the aiming point for the anterior screw), and the inferior pillar (the aiming point of the inferior screw) [27–29]. The three-column concept, introduced by Humphrey et al. [30] several years ago, is particularly useful when using a baseplate with variable-angle locking screws. However, in abnormal glenoids, a significant reduction in the surface area available for screw fixation occurs with different patterns depending on the erosion sites [7, 31].

4.4 Addressing Glenoid Bone Loss

Operative options for addressing glenoid bone loss include asymmetric reaming, the use of lateralized implants or augmented baseplates, and bone grafting using a bony-increased offset system. The surgeon's choice may depend on the amount of glenoid bone stock available, the severity of glenoid wear, and retroversion. Failure to address superior bone loss (i.e., Favard type E2/E3) can lead to superior tilt of the baseplate, scapular impingement, instability, inferior notching, and early loosening. A minor degree of posterior glenoid wear can be addressed with eccentric glenoid reaming, whereas bone grafting and augmented baseplates allow for the correction of greater amounts of glenoid wear and retroversion while preserving glenoid bone stock [32, 33]. Eccentric reaming, in cases of significant retroversion, results in less native bone available as structural support for the glenoid component and consequently increases the risk of vault perforation by the fixation peg [34]. Augmented glenoid components with wedges are commonly used to correct posterior and superior glenoid wear and to optimize version, inclination, and lateralization. Failure to correct glenoid retroversion can lead to eccentric loading and early loosening of the glenoid implant as well as reduced external rotation and posterior scapular notching. Augmented baseplates can have either a full wedge, half wedge, or a purely lateralized design. These implants include an additional metal augment that matches the glenoid bone defect without the need for excessive eccentric reaming or bone grafting. The use of augmented wedged glenoids also reduces the volume of bone removal, allowing for more cortical bone support of glenoid implants [35, 36]. Although there is limited literature available on clinical outcomes and only the short- to mid-term results are reported, the use of augmented baseplates has been found to enhance the stability of the construct when compared to a nonaugmented baseplate in the presence of large glenoid defects [37]. Furthermore, arthritic shoulders are often associated with posterior humeral head subluxation and joint line medialization caused by significant glenoid retroversion deformities. Excessive medialization of the joint line should be corrected: a lateralized center of rotation leads to decreased risk of scapular notching and instability of the implant as well as an improved rotational range of motion. Boileau et al. have described the bony increased-offset RSA technique (BIO-RSA) in order to produce a lateralized center of rotation and address glenoid bone loss. In this procedure, a bone graft is harvested from the humeral head and impacted between the baseplate and the native glenoid. The autograft may be symmetrical or asymmetrical (angled BIO-RSA) depending on the different glenoid bone defect that has to be filled. The technique allows the restoration of glenoid bone stock by correcting the baseplate version and inclination with the use of a graft with a trapezoidal shape while the COR is lateralized [38, 39]. Although there are some validated technical recommendations to optimize outcomes in RSA (e.g., the inferior overhang of the glenosphere, the lateralization of the center of rotation), still no consensus has been found regarding baseplate version and inclination and a minimum threshold value to be achieved for lateralization [40].

4.5 Lateralization

The term "lateralization" refers to the position of the center of rotation (COR) being lateral relative to the classic medialized design of reverse TSA. Excessive medialization of the COR caused by failure to restore the glenoid bone stock can lead to decreased motion and strength, reduced deltoid wrapping, and increased risk of instability due to impingement with the scapular lateral pillar. Medialization of the COR created by reaming the glenoid can be compensated and corrected with a lateralized prosthetic system [21]. Lateralization aims to obtain better stability of the construct by optimizing deltoid wrapping and compressive forces of the residual rotator cuff tendons when still present. Furthermore, it leads to higher compressive forces across the implant, thereby increasing its stability [41]. Lateralization on the glenoid side can occur at the baseplate, at the glenosphere, or through a bone graft (BIO-RSA). A lateralized baseplate reduces impingement increasing the shoulder's range of motion by minimizing scapular notching. The lateralization of the implant's COR increases the overall joint contact forces between the glenosphere and the scapula, with compression being the dominant component, while a minor increase is also observed in anteroposterior and superoinferior shear forces. As the COR is lateralized, the deltoid wrapping around the humerus increases, leading to decreased deltoid moment arm and a higher deltoid force required for abduction. While compression forces should improve implant stability, shear forces and bending moments increase the risk of glenoid loosening [42]. Another possible drawback of baseplate lateralization is the increased risk of scapular spine and acromial fractures caused by higher acromial stress [43]. Therefore, it is reasonable to consider that the surgery should aim to restore a degree of lateralization such as before the bony erosion due to osteoarthritis.

Humeral side lateralization can be achieved by various means. The stem may be curved instead of straight, the humeral tray position can be changed from "inlay" to "onlay," and the neck-shaft angle (NSA) can be modified from 155° to 145° or 135°. Humeral lateralization restores the position of tuberosities compared to Grammont's original design, leading to higher compressive joint reaction forces, increased stability, and increased deltoid tension and wrapping. Most recently, implants with NSA of 135° and 145° have been used combined with metallic lateralized baseplates and an "onlay" polyethylene insert in order to reduce the risk of scapular notching and to increase construct stability and shoulder ROM [44]. However, the ideal amount of global lateralization and whether the effective contribution comes from the glenoid or the humeral side remains unclear. They probably depend on patient anatomy, the quality of the remaining cuff and deltoid, and the amount of distalization of the humerus [45]. Some studies suggest that a lateralized COR of the glenosphere and 135° NSA could be more relevant for clinical outcomes rather than the humeral tray inlay/onlay position [46].

4.6 Preoperative Planning

Preoperative planning has become a critical step for shoulder arthroplasty. The advent of CT-based preoperative planning software has revolutionized surgeons' approach: access to three-dimensional (3D) models of the glenoid and the entire scapula allows for automatic measurements of the version and inclination, enhancing the understanding of the initial pathology, the deformities to be corrected, and consequently, the optimal positioning of the glenoid component in RSA.

Measurement techniques based on CT scan may be classified as either 2D, corrected 2D, or 3D techniques. 2D measurements are subject to variation based on patient positioning within the scanner. This is overcome in corrected 2D measurement by reorienting the imaging planes to the anatomical plane of the scapula using three landmarks: the junction of the scapular spine and the medial scapular margin, the center of the glenoid face, and the inferior tip of the scapula (Fig. 4.7).

The corrected coronal plane passes through all three of these points. The corrected axial plane is perpendicular to the corrected coronal plane and passes through the junction of the scapular spine and the medial scapular margin and the center of the glenoid. The corrected sagittal plane is perpendicular to both the corrected coronal and corrected axial planes. In this way, by correcting the imaging planes based on scapular anatomic references, the measurements are less affected by patient positioning within the scanner. 3D measurement techniques, on the other hand, rely on the manipulation of structures in three-dimensional space. 3D measures of the glenoid have been developed, such as the "Volumetric vault method" for quantifying bone stock, "the fitted-sphere method" for measuring glenoid orientation, and

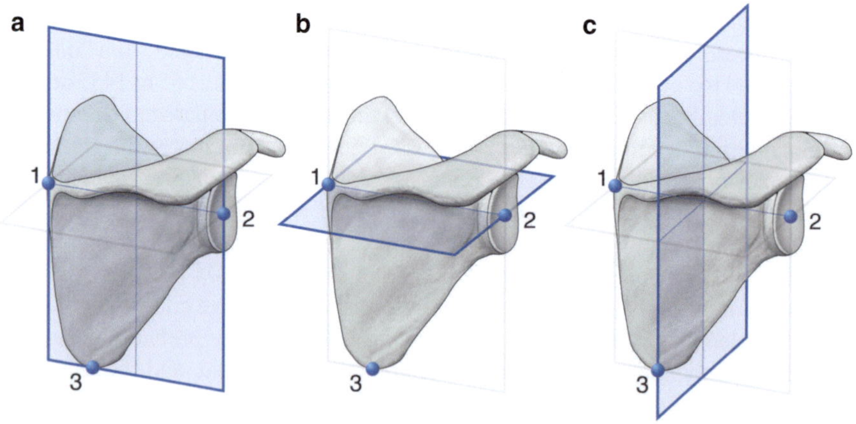

Fig. 4.7 Anatomic planes of the scapula. Three reference points are used to define the anatomic planes of the scapula: (1) the junction of the scapular spine with the medial margin of the scapula, (2) the center of the glenoid, and (3) the inferior tip of the scapula. The corrected coronal plane passes through all three of these points (**a**). The corrected axial plane (**b**) is perpendicular to the corrected coronal plane and passes through points (1) and (2). The corrected sagittal plane (**c**) is perpendicular to both the corrected coronal and axial planes

surface area measures of glenoid biconcavity. These methods use a spherical surface fitted to the glenoid face. The orientation of the glenoid face in three dimensions is given by the radial ray from the center of the fitted sphere to the center of the glenoid. The projection of this radial ray into the corrected axial and coronal planes gives version and inclination, respectively. Regarding the calculation of the bone stock, on the other hand, this method requires further implementation.

Corrected 2D measurements generally remain the most practical metrics. Oblique multiplanar reconstruction tools are widely available on standard PACS and advanced visualization systems and allow users to quickly reorient images to the anatomic planes of the scapula.

There are two different 3D planning systems: semiautomated systems and fully automated volumetry-based systems. In semiautomated systems, Digital Imaging and Communications in Medicine (DICOM) CT scans are uploaded into the online planning software. The study is manually segmented by engineers of the manufacturer to reconstruct the shoulder in a 3D model for preoperative planning. The humerus is subtracted, and landmarks are identified on the scapula to include the scapula trigonum, the inferior angle, and the center of the glenoid to determine the plane of the scapula and the transverse scapula line. The plane of the glenoid is then determined by placing three landmarks on the glenoid fossa. Glenoid version and inclination are then calculated based on these measurements. In automated software, voxels specific to the scapula are isolated using image recognition technology without manual engineer input. A best-fit plane is then defined using these voxels to define the plane of the scapula, and similarly, a best-fit sphere is defined to determine the glenoid rim. Version and inclination are then automatically calculated by using the software and by comparing the best-fit plane of the glenoid to the horizontal and vertical planes of the scapula.

After reconstruction, the virtual 3D model is ready for planning into the preoperative application. Before starting, the surgeon must validate the reconstruction using landmarks and references, some of these landmarks will be asked to be located intraoperative afterward in case of navigated procedure. During the planning, it is possible to choose the dimension of the baseplate, its position, and the use of augments to reduce or to increase the version and inclination. The software generates colored and numeric feedback according to matching between the bony glenoid and the prosthetic baseplate, about the position of the baseplate (version, height, anteroposterior translation), and medialization or lateralization of the center of rotation (with respect to the normal center of rotation and bony landmarks useful in RSA). Position can be regulated by degree per degree and millimeter per millimeter (Figs. 4.8 and 4.9).

It is recommended to rotate the virtual 3D scapula model on all planes and axes to ensure the position of the baseplate with respect to the peg as well. In addition, a 2D check should be performed in order to ensure the complete insertion of the peg inside the bone without perforating or touching the cortices of the scapular neck to improve stability and reduce the risk of perioperative fracture. During the virtual positioning of the metaglene, surgeons can evaluate the correct seating of the glenoid component and how much bone has to be removed from the articular surface.

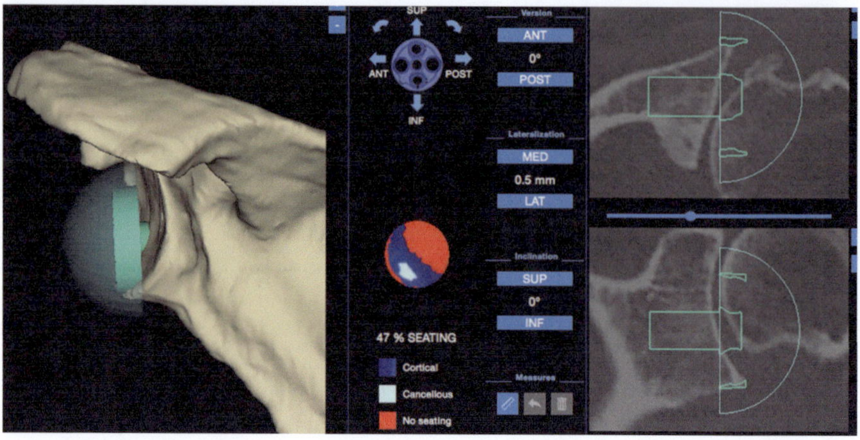

Fig. 4.8 Preoperative planning with the software "Blueprint" (Stryker). Reproduced with permission by Stryker

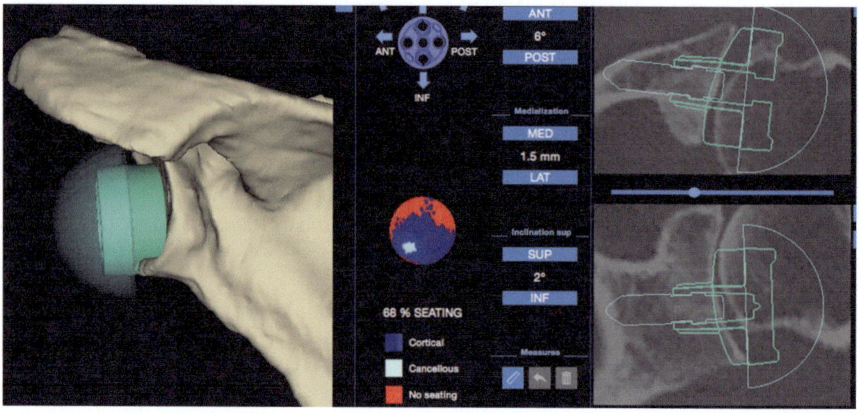

Fig. 4.9 Preoperative planning with the software "Blueprint" (Stryker) with glenoid augmentation used to correct the glenoid bone loss and increase the percentage of seating of the glenoid component. Reproduced with permission by Stryker

Desired bone–prosthesis contact is more than 90% of the baseplate. After that, some of the software give the opportunity to direct the screws to obtain maximal screw length into the bone without exiting the cortices [47] excessively (Fig. 4.10).

Berhouet et al. [40] did a comparative RSA preoperative planning study and found a strong agreement between surgeons on the placement of the glenoid preparation guide pin. Conversely, there was little consensus on the criteria for the lateralization, version, and inclination of the glenoid baseplate for RSA. This may be due to the current lack of recommendations in the literature for glenoid reaming and glenoid lateralization.

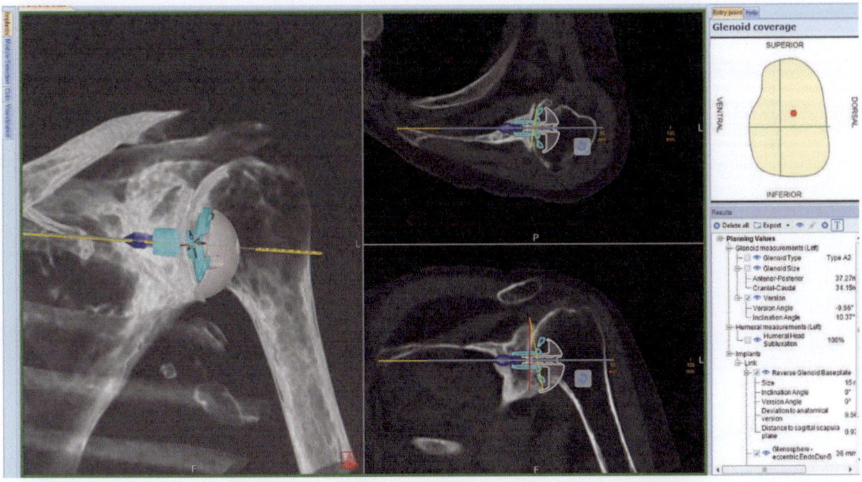

Fig. 4.10 Preoperative planning with the software "MediCAD." Reproduced with permission by MediCAD

Nevertheless, 3D information from preoperative planning seems beneficial for assessing the pathologic glenoid deformity and to limit its impact on the baseplate position achieved by different surgeons.

Planning systems can help surgeons only during the preoperative phase without granting real-time assistance during the intraoperative phase. Therefore, surgeons showed increasing interest in the application of new technologies in the RSA world such as patient-specific implants, computer-assisted intraoperative navigation, and augmented reality [48].

4.7 Patient-Specific Instrumentation (PSI)

Preoperative planning with dedicated software is the first step for manufacturing patient-specific instrumentation (Fig. 4.11). Following the same procedure, once the surgeon is satisfied with the implant position and orientation, the software generates a patient-specific surgical guide model, allowing for a final check. This guide model is then saved and used for rapid prototyping. The process of planning and creating the guide's computer model can take up to 15 min based on the user's experience and the patient's anatomy. The guide automatically created by the software has a central cylinder with a hole that orientates guide pin insertion during operation. This central cylinder hole is precisely located and angled according to the surgeon-defined entry point. The rest of the guide consists of a body that provides sufficient surface area to sit firmly on the glenoid surface using the coracoid base as a reference [49].

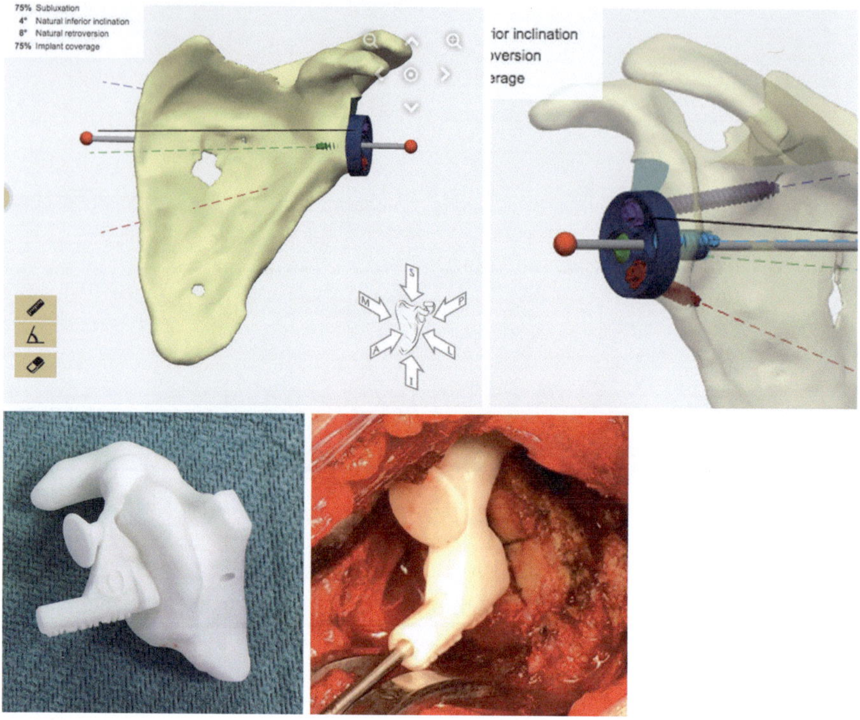

Fig. 4.11 Preoperative planning with software "Trumatch" (DePuy) and intraoperative view of central pin positioning using PSI. Reproduced with permission by DePuy

Most of all available published articles using PSI for shoulder arthroplasty (90.9%) reported mean postoperative version and inclination errors of 5° or less compared with preoperative plans.

However, despite the differences between PSI and standard instrumentation found in most individual studies, a meta-analysis of Cabarcas et al. [50] revealed significant heterogeneity in study methodologies and no statistically significant differences in version error, inclination error, or positional offset between PSI and standard instrumentation. One possible explanation for the lack of significant differences in accuracy between PSI and standard instrumentation is the operative experience of senior surgeons. Several senior surgeons who were involved in these studies regularly perform shoulder arthroplasties at particularly high volumes. Because of increased operative experience, they may have had higher accuracy and reduced variability with standard instrumentation. Thus, the discrepancy between PSI and standard instrumentation may have been reduced in their hands. The study by Iannotti et al. found that implantation accuracy was significantly impacted by surgeon expertise when using PSI, with the less experienced surgeon producing more accurate results. This finding suggests that PSI can be particularly advantageous for novice or low-volume shoulder surgeons [50].

4.8 Navigation

The next step in the utilizing 3D anatomical information is to move from planning to preoperative application. A navigated procedure offers a connection between preoperative planning and the intraoperative phase, leading surgeons to better understand and treat glenoid deformities. The preoperative planning is uploaded to the intraoperative application, and the patient's data are checked. The navigation system hardware consists of a platform positioned in a sterile fashion at patient's feet and tracker-equipped surgical instruments. Primarily, the optical navigation trackers are registered and calibrated on the computer. Then, threaded screws are positioned into the inferolateral surface at the base of the coracoid process to secure the scapular tracker. The tracker must remain stable and not loosen during surgery as it serves as the reference for all the procedure; otherwise, the navigation system will not be accurate. Anatomic landmarks (anterior and posterior surface and baseline of the coracoid process; superior, inferior, anterior, and posterior margins of the glenoid surface; anterior, inferior, and posterior rim lines of the glenoid, anterior, and inferior neckline) are registered with a handheld tracker to check and superimpose the patient's scapula with the CT-based model. Colored feedback confirms the matching of the registered data with the patient's CT-based anatomy (green: perfect match; yellow: acceptable coupling, red: unacceptable registration). Then the preoperative planning is shown on the screen of the platform. Surgeons can now prepare the glenoid, step-by-step, as in conventional technique, but with the use of tracker-equipped instruments and guided by the 2D and 3D feedback on the screen to achieve the preoperative planning [47].

4.9 Mixed Reality

Another new innovative technology is mixed-reality-guided implantation, a form of augmented reality that involves the use of a headset that projects a virtual 3D reconstruction, in the form of a hologram, of the scapula that can be manually positioned by the surgeon.

In this way, the surgeon can access computer-based solutions in real-time during the procedure while remaining complete sterile to access 3D holograms related to the patient imaging and enabling remote interaction with colleagues located outside the operating room [51].

Patient scapula 3D reconstruction extracted from her CT scan, the planning of the positioning of the glenoid, and the whole operative technique developed in 3D holograms were transmitted into his operating headset in real-time during the intervention. CT scan scapula reconstruction can be overlapped on the visible part of the bone with manual adjustment by simple gestures in front of the headset. Hence, the surgeon was able to compare, stage-by-stage, what he was doing with what had to be done. Although it is only in its infancy, this technology has immense potential for future surgeons as a practical and educational tool.

Take Home Messages

1. Preoperative planning on a CT scan is a fundamental step before surgery: many software has been developed by different companies with its pros and cons.
2. Nowadays, there is still no perfect planning: there are many theoretical questions about what the corrective standards should be to obtain the best biomechanics and many aspects have not yet been explored and should be taken into consideration.
3. Applying the digital planning to the actual surgery is still a crucial point: many devices and systems have been developed to achieve this: PSI, navigation, and mixed reality.

References

1. Walch G, Badet R, Boulahia A, Khoury A. Morphologic study of the glenoid in primary glenohumeral osteoarthritis. J Arthroplast. 1999;14:756–60.
2. Bercik MJ, et al. A modification to the Walch classification of the glenoid in primary glenohumeral osteoarthritis using three-dimensional imaging. J Shoulder Elb Surg. 2016;25:1601–6.
3. Lo L, et al. Glenoid bony morphology of osteoarthritis prior to shoulder arthroplasty: what the surgeon wants to know and why. Skeletal Radiol. 2021;50:881–94.
4. Favard L, Berhouet J, Walch G, Chaoui J, Lévigne C. Superiore Glenoidinklination und glenoidaler Knochenverlust: Definition, Assessment, biomechanische Konsequenzen und operative Optionen. Orthopade. 2017;46:1015–21.
5. Bryce CD, et al. Two-dimensional glenoid version measurements vary with coronal and sagittal scapular rotation. J Bone Joint Surg Am. 2010;92:692–9.
6. Kwon YW, Powell KA, Yum JK, Brems JJ, Iannotti JP. Use of three-dimensional computed tomography for the analysis of the glenoid anatomy. J Shoulder Elb Surg. 2005;14:85–90.
7. Frankle MA, Teramoto A, Luo ZP, Levy JC, Pupello D. Glenoid morphology in reverse shoulder arthroplasty: classification and surgical implications. J Shoulder Elb Surg. 2009;18:874–85.
8. Plessers K, et al. Automated quantification of glenoid bone defects using 3-dimensional measurements. J Shoulder Elb Surg. 2020;29:1050–8.
9. Walch G, Vezeridis PS, Boileau P, Deransart P, Chaoui J. Three-dimensional planning and use of patient-specific guides improve glenoid component position: an in vitro study. J Shoulder Elb Surg. 2015;24:302–9.
10. Seidl AJ, Williams GR, Boileau P. Challenges in reverse shoulder arthroplasty: addressing glenoid bone loss. Orthopedics. 2016;39:14–23.
11. Keener JD, Patterson BM, Orvets N, Aleem AW, Chamberlain AM. Optimizing reverse shoulder arthroplasty component position in the setting of advanced arthritis with posterior glenoid erosion: a computer-enhanced range of motion analysis. J Shoulder Elb Surg. 2018;27:339–49.
12. Strauss EJ, Roche C, Flurin PH, Wright T, Zuckerman JD. The glenoid in shoulder arthroplasty. J Shoulder Elb Surg. 2009;18:819–33.
13. Van de Bunt F, Pearl ML, Lee EK, Peng L, Didomenico P. Glenoid version by CT scan: an analysis of clinical measurement error and introduction of a protocol to reduce variability. Skeletal Radiol. 2015;44:1627–35.
14. Fulin P, et al. Study of the variability of scapular inclination and the glenoid version – considerations for preoperative planning: clinical-radiological study. BMC Musculoskelet Disord. 2017;18:1–7.
15. Matsumura N, et al. Morphologic features of humeral head and glenoid version in the normal glenohumeral joint. J Shoulder Elb Surg. 2014;23:1724–30.

16. Hsu JE, Ricchetti ET, Huffman GR, Iannotti JP, Glaser DL. Addressing glenoid bone deficiency and asymmetric posterior erosion in shoulder arthroplasty. J Shoulder Elb Surg. 2013;22:1298–308.
17. Chan K, et al. Characterization of the Walch B3 glenoid in primary osteoarthritis. J Shoulder Elb Surg. 2017;26:909–14.
18. Maurer A, et al. Assessment of glenoid inclination on routine clinical radiographs and computed tomography examinations of the shoulder. J Shoulder Elb Surg. 2012;21:1096–103.
19. Churchill RS, Brems JJ, Kotschi H. Glenoid size, inclination, and version: an anatomic study. J Shoulder Elb Surg. 2001;10:327–32.
20. Boileau P, et al. The reverse shoulder arthroplasty angle: a new measurement of glenoid inclination for reverse shoulder arthroplasty. J Shoulder Elb Surg. 2019;28:1281–90.
21. Laver L, Garrigues GE. Avoiding superior tilt in reverse shoulder arthroplasty: a review of the literature and technical recommendations. J Shoulder Elb Surg. 2014;23:1582–90.
22. Randelli P, et al. Optimal glenoid component inclination in reverse shoulder arthroplasty. How to improve implant stability. Musculoskelet Surg. 2014;98:15–8.
23. Gutiérrez S, Walker M, Willis M, Pupello DR, Frankle MA. Effects of tilt and glenosphere eccentricity on baseplate/bone interface forces in a computational model, validated by a mechanical model, of reverse shoulder arthroplasty. J Shoulder Elb Surg. 2011;20:732–9.
24. Edwards TB, et al. Inferior tilt of the glenoid component does not decrease scapular notching in reverse shoulder arthroplasty: results of a prospective randomized study. J Shoulder Elb Surg. 2012;21:641–6.
25. Simovitch RW, Zumstein MA, Lohri E, Helmy N, Gerber C. Predictors of scapular notching in patients managed with the delta III reverse total shoulder replacement. J Bone Joint Surg Am. 2007;89:588–600.
26. Eyberg BA, et al. Identifying areas of screw fixation in glenoids with severe bone loss in shoulder arthroplasty. J Shoulder Elb Surg. 2022;31:S136–42.
27. Kelly JD, Humphrey CS, Norris TR. Optimizing glenosphere position and fixation in reverse shoulder arthroplasty, Part One: the twelve-mm rule. J Shoulder Elb Surg. 2008;17:589–94.
28. Stephens BF, Hebert CT, Azar FM, Mihalko WM, Throckmorton TW. Optimal baseplate rotational alignment for locking-screw fixation in reverse total shoulder arthroplasty: a three-dimensional computer-aided design study. J Shoulder Elb Surg. 2015;24:1367–71.
29. Karelse A, Kegels L, De Wilde L. The pillars of the scapula. Clin Anat. 2007;20:392–9.
30. Humphrey CS, Kelly JD, Norris TR. Optimizing glenosphere position and fixation in reverse shoulder arthroplasty, Part Two: the three-column concept. J Shoulder Elb Surg. 2008;17:595–601.
31. DiStefano JG, et al. Optimal screw placement for base plate fixation in reverse total shoulder arthroplasty. J Shoulder Elb Surg. 2011;20:467–76.
32. Virk M, et al. Clinical and radiographic outcomes with a posteriorly augmented glenoid for Walch B2, B3, and C glenoids in reverse total shoulder arthroplasty. J Shoulder Elb Surg. 2020;29:e196–204.
33. Kersten AD, Flores-Hernandez C, Hoenecke HR, D'Lima DD. Posterior augmented glenoid designs preserve more bone in biconcave glenoids. J Shoulder Elb Surg. 2015;24:1135–41.
34. Hermida JC, Flores-Hernandez C, Hoenecke HR, D'Lima DD. Augmented wedge-shaped glenoid component for the correction of glenoid retroversion: a finite element analysis. J Shoulder Elb Surg. 2014;23:347–54.
35. Abdic S, Lockhart J, Alnusif N, Johnson JA, Athwal GS. Glenoid baseplate screw fixation in reverse shoulder arthroplasty: does locking screw position and orientation matter? J Shoulder Elb Surg. 2021;30:1207–13.
36. Allred JJ, Flores-Hernandez C, Hoenecke HR, D'Lima DD. Posterior augmented glenoid implants require less bone removal and generate lower stresses: a finite element analysis. J Shoulder Elb Surg. 2016;25:823–30.
37. Martin EJ, Duquin TR, Ehrensberger MT. Reverse total shoulder arthroplasty baseplate stability in superior bone loss with augmented implant. J Shoulder Elb Arthroplast. 2021;5:247154922110206.

38. Mourad W, Wiater JM, Wiater BP, Martusiewicz A. Baseplate options for reverse total shoulder arthroplasty. Curr Rev Musculoskelet Med. 2020;13:769–75.
39. Boileau P, et al. Angled BIO-RSA (bony-increased offset–reverse shoulder arthroplasty): a solution for the management of glenoid bone loss and erosion. J Shoulder Elb Surg. 2017;26:2133–42.
40. Berhouet J, et al. Preoperative planning of baseplate position in reverse shoulder arthroplasty: still no consensus on lateralization, version and inclination. Orthop Traumatol Surg Res. 2022;108:103115.
41. Costantini O, Choi DS, Kontaxis A, Gulotta LV. The effects of progressive lateralization of the joint center of rotation of reverse total shoulder implants. J Shoulder Elb Surg. 2015;24:1120–8.
42. Eno JJT, et al. The biomechanics of subscapularis repair in reverse shoulder arthroplasty: the effect of lateralization and insertion site. J Orthop Res. 2020;38:888–94.
43. Bauer S, Corbaz J, Athwal GS, Walch G, Blakeney WG. Lateralization in reverse shoulder arthroplasty. J Clin Med. 2021;10:1–14.
44. Valenti P, Sekri J, Kany J, Nidtahar I, Werthel JD. Benefits of a metallic lateralized baseplate prolonged by a long metallic post in reverse shoulder arthroplasty to address glenoid bone loss. Int Orthop. 2019;43:2131–9.
45. Werthel JD, et al. Lateralization in reverse shoulder arthroplasty: a descriptive analysis of different implants in current practice. Int Orthop. 2019;43:2349–60.
46. Meshram P, Joseph J, Zhou Y, Srikumaran U, McFarland EG. Lateralized glenosphere reverse shoulder arthroplasty: inlay and onlay designs have similar clinical outcomes in patients with glenohumeral osteoarthritis. J Shoulder Elb Surg. 2022;31:747–54.
47. Moreschini F, et al. Preoperative CT-based planning integrated with intra-operative navigation in reverse shoulder arthroplasty: data acquisition and analysis protocol, and preliminary results of navigated versus conventional surgery. Dose-Response. 2020;18:1–11.
48. Giorgini A, Tarallo L, Novi M, Porcellini G. Computer-assisted surgery in reverse shoulder arthroplasty: early experience. Indian J Orthop. 2021;55:1003–8.
49. Mohammad Sadeghi M, et al. Three dimensional patient-specific guides for guide pin positioning in reverse shoulder arthroplasty: an experimental study on different glenoid types. J Orthop Surg. 2022;30:10225536221079432.
50. Cabarcas BC, et al. Accuracy of patient-specific instrumentation in shoulder arthroplasty: a systematic review and meta-analysis. JSES Open Access. 2019;3:117–29.
51. Gregory TM, Gregory J, Sledge J, Allard R, Mir O. Surgery guided by mixed reality: presentation of a proof of concept. Acta Orthop. 2018;89:480–3.

Part II

Elbow Arthroplasty

E. Guerra

Patient Position and General Setting in Elbow Arthroplasty

5

F. Coliva, A. Sessa, M. Monetta, A. Ritali, G. Carbone, and E. Guerra

5.1 Introduction

Elbow arthroplasty is currently indicated in primary and secondary osteoarthritis or non-reducible fractures [1, 2]. It is performed significantly less frequently than other arthroplasties [3], and it is a challenging procedure and has to be executed by expert elbow surgeons.

It can be performed with patients in different positions depending on their comorbidity or pathologies and the surgeon's and/or anesthetist's preferences. Elbow arthroplasty can be executed in any position described in this chapter. These setups will not interfere with the surgical approach (posterior, posteromedial, posterolateral approach) or the surgical technique.

We will describe the supine decubitus (SDP), prone decubitus (PDP), lateral decubitus position (LDP), and their respective room setups, and we will try to clarify the advantages and disadvantages of every single setting.

5.2 Supine Decubitus Position (SDP)

The supine position is probably the most convenient setup. The patient is placed supine on the operating table with the affected arm positioned at 90° of anterior flexion and the elbow flexed to 90° [4] so that the operative arm is positioned above the chest (Fig. 5.1). A sterile tourniquet can be used to avoid surgical field contamination [5] and to maximize the exposure of the operative field.

Surgical sterile towels can be used to maintain the elbow at 90° flexion without interfering with endotracheal intubation [6]. Additionally, a surgical assistant is

F. Coliva · A. Sessa · M. Monetta · A. Ritali · G. Carbone · E. Guerra (✉)
Shoulder and Elbow Unit – IRCCS, Istituto Ortopedico Rizzoli, Bologna, Italy
e-mail: enrico.guerra@ior.it

G. M. Marcheggiani Muccioli et al. (eds.), *Easy Planning in Elective Primary Orthopedic Procedures*, https://doi.org/10.1007/978-3-031-77006-7_5

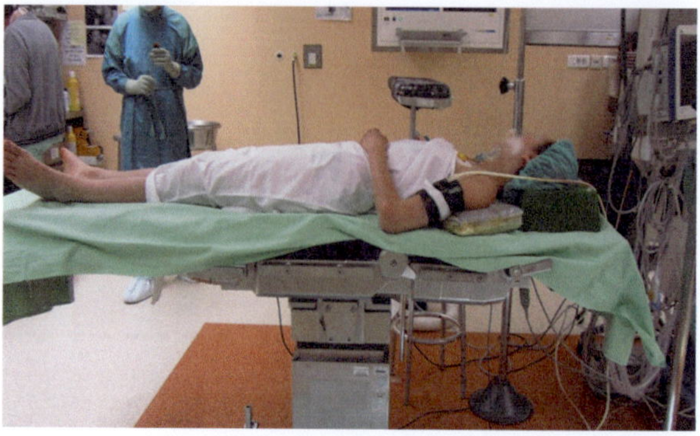

Fig. 5.1 Supine position with the patient placed in the middle of the operating table and the tourniquet placed on the affected arm

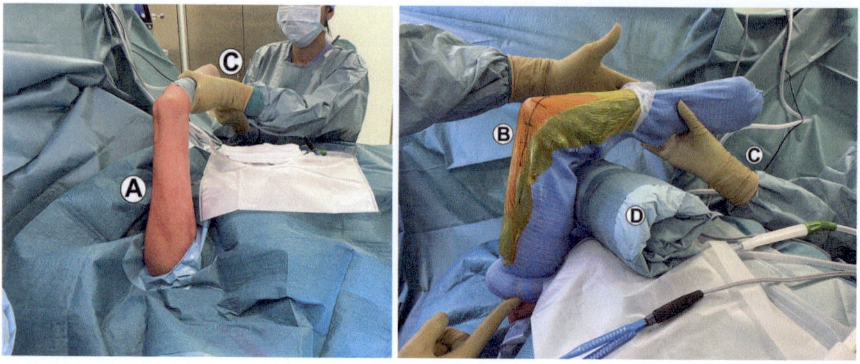

Fig. 5.2 and 5.3 Elbow in surgical position before (A) and after (B) sterile draping and positioning of the sterile tourniquet. The help of a surgical assistant (C) is needed to achieve the maximum mobility of the elbow, sterile towels (D) can be used to stabilize the position

required on the contralateral side of the table to hold the arm, allowing for easy adjustments of elbow flexion–extension and forearm pronation–supination, thereby maximizing elbow mobility (Figs. 5.2 and 5.3). On the other hand, the main disadvantage of this position is the need for an assistant to maintain proper elbow positioning. Alternatively, a Lyoid–Davis leg support, a mechanical arm holder attached at the level of the contralateral shoulder, or a padded L-bar placed on the ipsilateral side of the table can be used if greater elbow flexion is required [7]. These devices allow the maintenance of a firm position but at the same time limit elbow movement.

The advantages of the SDP are both for the orthopedic surgeon and for the anesthetist: this position allows the surgeon to obtain maximum degrees of flexion/extension or prono-supination of the elbow, providing optimal exposure of anatomical structures, such as the humeral and ulnar canals [6]. At the same time, the supine position is preferred by anesthesiologists as it provides the easiest access to the patient's face and upper respiratory airways. This position is also ideal for patients with multiple fractures due to high-energy trauma, especially if the spine is also involved [7]. At our institution, SDP is the proferred choice for treating patients with either primary or secondary osteoarthritis for the easy and fast setup and for the wide mobility of the elbow.

The main complications associated with the SDP are related to the positioning of the head and the shoulder. Excessive traction on the brachial plexus is generated by the abduction of the arm over 90°, lateral head rotation toward the contralateral side, or pronation of the arm. Although none of these positions are required for elbow arthroplasty, they should be avoided as a general rule [8].

5.3 Lateral Decubitus Position (LDP)

The LDP is more challenging to set up than the SDP. This position is less commonly used in orthopedic surgery than the supine one, so it is crucial that the entire operating room team is expert to reduce the risk of complications and the time required to set up.

The patient is placed lying on the contralateral side with the affected arm placed at 90° of anterior flexion and 90°of internal rotation of the shoulder [4]. The elbow is placed over a support, which must be placed 3–4 cm proximal to the cubital fossa to interfere with flexion as little as possible, leaving room for the joint to be manipulated as requested. A non-sterile tourniquet can be applied if it does not interfere with the surgical field; in smaller patients, we recommend using a sterile tourniquet and placing it as proximally as possible [4], for the same reasons discussed in the section on the SDP (Fig. 5.4 and 5.5).

We suggest placing the contralateral arm at 90° of anterior flexion of the shoulder and 90°of elbow flexion with the hand in front of the patient's face [4]. Some authors suggest using an arm sling for the contralateral arm for safe positioning [9]. It is important to place padding between the legs to prevent common peroneal and saphenous nerve injury [8] and beneath the scapula to protect bone prominence.

To maintain a firm LDP, we suggest using a vacuum beanbag placed under the patient's axilla in order to avoid interference with arm positioning and intubation for anesthesia, as shown in Fig. 5.4. It is important to prevent axillary compression to avoid brachial plexus injuries, for this, an axillary roll can be used [10].

At our institution, we usually perform LDP in patients with complex distal humerus fractures. Our first choice in these cases is to attempt fracture reduction and fixation when possible, and the LDP provides great stability to the distal humerus, allowing the surgeon to manage the fracture segments in the most stable position. If the fracture turns out to be non-reducible, we are prepared to perform elbow arthroplasty in the same setting. With this position, there is no need for a surgical assistant to mantain the arm in the correct position through the procedure. However the range of elbow flexion may be limited [6]. LDP might not be ideal for patients with respiratory issues since the dependent lung is relatively underventilated and overperfused, while the nondependent lung is overventilated and underperfused [8]. The head should be well secured in a neutral position to avoid ocular damage and brachial plexus complications [8, 10]. Other complications, such as

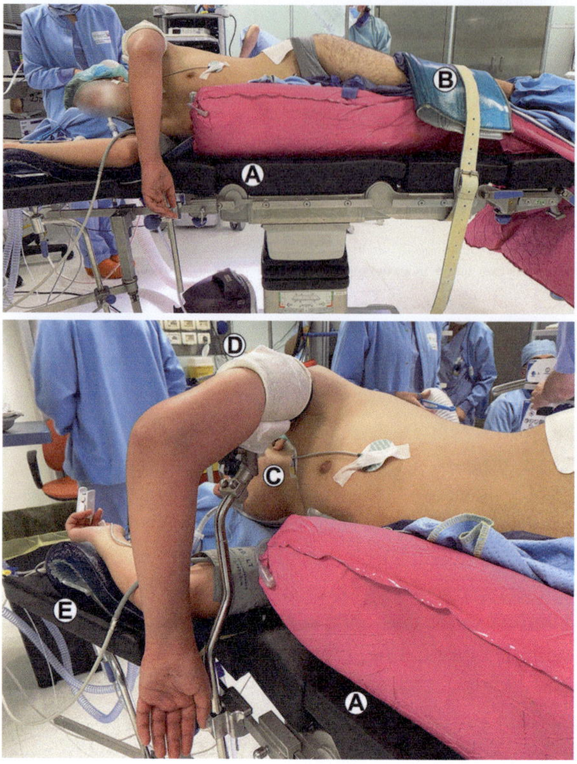

Fig. 5.4 and 5.5 Patient positioning for lateral position. The vacuum beanbag (A) is placed under the patient's axilla and a belt-and-padding (B) is placed around the patient's knees to improve stabilization and avoid compression injuries. The affected arm is placed over a specific support (C) and the tourniquet (D) has to be placed as proximal as possible. The contralateral arm (E) is placed as shown

contralateral deltoid compartment syndrome, have been described in an anabolic steroid abusers [11].

5.4 Prone Decubitus Position (PDP)

Prone decubitus position (PDP) is less frequently used for elbow arthroplasty worldwide, and is rarely employed at our institution.

This positioning is mainly used in spinal surgery, but it can also be used to reach the posterior aspect of extremities if needed. In order to position the patient correctly without risking injuries, three or four assistants are needed: head and neck should be maintained in a neutral position by one person throughout the entire positioning process, while the others slowly rotate the patient from supine to lateral and then to prone decubitus, keeping the arms at the sides during the entire maneuver [10]. This procedure must be performed safely to avoid iatrogenic injuries, which are particularly likely in anesthetized patients [12, 13]. If surgery is performed for fractures, always keep the affected side as the upper extremity while rotating the patient. Sliding sheets or a sliding board might be helpful during this procedure [14].

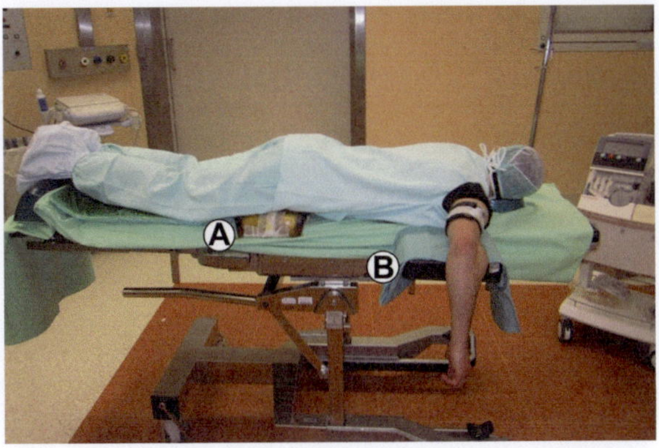

Fig. 5.6 Patient positioning for prone position. Padded rolls (A) are used to preserve bony prominences. Elbow stability is given by support placed on the table side as shown (B)

Ventilation must be preserved by placing padded rolls under the thorax and pelvis; bony prominences must also be preserved (Fig. 5.6) [10]. The patient should be placed with 10–15° of reverse Trendelenburg to decrease intraocular pressure and facial edema [15].

The patient's shoulder has to be placed at a maximum 90° of adduction to avoid brachial plexus damage and should rest slightly lower than the level of the table [10].

This operating table setup and patient positioning help the surgeon by providing greater stability to the elbow and reducing the risk of neurovascular lesions [16, 17]. On the other side, PDP has to be avoided in patients with eye diseases and cardiac issues [18].

Take Home Messages

1. Our suggestion is to use supine decubitus position (SDP) for elbow arthroplasties due to primary or secondary osteoarthritis and to prefer the lateral decubitus position (LDP) for complex fractures where a prosthetic solution cannot be escluded.
2. Work in your comfort zone: the best position is always the one you are more familiar with.
3. Decide together with the anesthetist which position is better for the patient.

References

1. Kumar S, Mahanta S. Primary total elbow arthroplasty. Indian J Orthop. 2013;47(6):608–14. https://doi.org/10.4103/0019-5413.121592.
2. Page BJ, Lee BM. Total elbow arthroplasty for distal humerus fractures. J Orthop Trauma. 2020;34(2):S7–8. https://doi.org/10.1097/BOT.0000000000001821.
3. Zhou H, Orvets ND, Merlin G, et al. Total elbow arthroplasty in the United States: evaluation of cost, patient demographics, and complication rates. Orthop Rev. 2016;8(1):6113. https://doi.org/10.4081/or.2016.6113.

4. Prkic A, de Vos MJ, Wagener ML, The B, Eygendaal D. Total elbow arthroplasty: why and how. JBJS Essent Surg Tech. 2017;7(1):e5. https://doi.org/10.2106/JBJS.ST.16.00087.
5. Rotini R, Ricciarelli M, Guerra E, Marinelli A, Celli A. Elbow hemiarthroplasty in distal humeral fractures: Indication, surgical technique and results. Injury. 2020:S0020138320309463. https://doi.org/10.1016/j.injury.2020.11.020. Published online November.
6. Horneff JG, Ramsey ML. Surgical exposures for total elbow arthroplasty. J Am Acad Orthop Surg. 2019;27(22):e986–94. https://doi.org/10.5435/JAAOS-D-17-00916.
7. Wijeratna M, Thomas S, Van Rensburg L. The supine position for elbow surgery. Ann R Coll Surg Engl. 2012;94(6):446. https://doi.org/10.1308/003588412X13373405386015n.
8. Knight DJ, Mahajan RP. Patient positioning in anaesthesia. Contin Educ Anaesth Crit Care Pain. 2004;4(5):160–3. https://doi.org/10.1093/bjaceaccp/mkh044.
9. Rammohan R, Matthews T. Novel use of an arm sling for safe positioning of the non-operative arm during upper limb surgery in the lateral decubitus position. Ann R Coll Surg Engl. 2020;102(3):238–9. https://doi.org/10.1308/rcsann.2020.0005.
10. Bonnaig N, Dailey S, Archdeacon M. Proper patient positioning and complication prevention in orthopaedic surgery. J Bone Jt Surg. 2014;96(13):1135–40. https://doi.org/10.2106/JBJS.M.01267.
11. Wijesuriya JD, Cowling PD, Izod C, Burton DJ. Deltoid compartment syndrome as a complication of lateral decubitus positioning for contralateral elbow surgery in an anabolic steroid abuser. Shoulder Elb. 2014;6(3):200–3. https://doi.org/10.1177/1758573214530607.
12. Gill B, Heavner JE. Postoperative visual loss associated with spine surgery. Eur Spine J. 2006;15(4):479–84. https://doi.org/10.1007/s00586-005-0914-6.
13. Edgcombe H, Carter K, Yarrow S. Anaesthesia in the prone position. Br J Anaesth. 2008;100(2):165–83. https://doi.org/10.1093/bja/aem380.
14. Bowers M. Prone positioning for surgery. J Perioper Pract. 2012;22(5):157–62. https://doi.org/10.1177/175045891202200504.
15. Hoski JJ, Eismont FJ, Green BA. Blindness as a complication of intraoperative positioning. A case report. J Bone Joint Surg Am. 1993;75(8):1231–2. https://doi.org/10.2106/00004623-199308000-00015.
16. Baker CL, Shalvoy RM. The prone position for elbow arthroscopy. Clin Sports Med. 1991;10(3):623–8.
17. De Pellegrin M, Fracassetti D, Moharamzadeh D, Origo C, Catena N. Advantages and disadvantages of the prone position in the surgical treatment of supracondylar humerus fractures in children. A literature review. Injury. 2018;49:S37–42. https://doi.org/10.1016/j.injury.2018.09.046.
18. Kwee MM, Ho YH, Rozen WM. The prone position during surgery and its complications: a systematic review and evidence-based guidelines. Int Surg. 2015;100(2):292–303. https://doi.org/10.9738/INTSURG-D-13-00256.1.

Planning in Total Elbow Arthroplasty

6

F. Tortorella, L. Ferra, A. Marinelli, C. Buondonno,
M. Cavallo, and E. Guerra

6.1 Introduction

Total elbow arthroplasty (TEA) is considered a rescue surgery for the elbow due to the functional limitation it imposes on the patient and the associated complications [1]. Before performing an elbow prosthesis, careful patient selection is mandatory, along with suitable surgical planning. Patients must be aware that this procedure requires good postoperative compliance, entails lifelong limitations, and arries the risk of major complications, such as infections or implant loosening, which might severely affect their quality of life. Indications for TEA are end-stage arthritis, chronic inflammatory arthropathies with gross instability and deformation of the articular surfaces, or complex and comminuted fractures of the distal humerus, in which reduction and fixation are not possible [2]. Due to the drawbacks of the elbow prosthesis procedure, young age is a contraindication, and patients are usually treated only if they are at least 65 years old.

Due to pathological changes in elbow anatomy, different types of implants may be chosen for replacement.

6.2 Types of Implants (Linked or Unlinked) and Surgical Indication

One of the key components in prosthetic design is the link mechanism between the humeral and the ulnar component. Over time, several different concepts have been developed and investigated, with drawbacks and positive aspects, leading to three main groups of implants.

F. Tortorella · L. Ferra · A. Marinelli · C. Buondonno · M. Cavallo · E. Guerra (✉)
Shoulder and Elbow Unit – IRCCS, Istituto Ortopedico Rizzoli, Bologna, Italy
e-mail: enrico.guerra@ior.it

G. M. Marcheggiani Muccioli et al. (eds.), *Easy Planning in Elective Primary Orthopedic Procedures*, https://doi.org/10.1007/978-3-031-77006-7_6

Constrained elbow arthroplasty employs a simple hinged mechanism with less than 1° varus–valgus laxity. This design provides high joint stability but also generates significant stress at the bone-cement and prosthesis-cement interfaces for both the humeral and ulnar components. Mid-to-long-term studies have revealed an unacceptably high rate of implant loosening requiring prosthetic revisions, leading to the abandonment of this mechanism in favor of newer designs.

Semi-constrained or "linked" implants were developed to overcome the high loosening rate of previous constrained designs. These models utilize a "loose" hinge mechanism, allowing for 7–10° varus–valgus laxity and 7–10° of axial rotation. This represented a significant advancement in prosthesis design: the implant retains intrinsic stability, allowing its use in cases of severe instability with capsular and ligament disruption. However, the slight laxity of the hinge system is sufficient to substantially reduce the incidence of aseptic loosening by minimizing the transmission of forces across the prosthetic stems [3]. To date, semi-constrained implants have completely replaced constrained designs for primary procedures.

Unlinked elbow arthroplasty (also referred to as "unhinged" or "resurfacing") completely relies on the patient's soft tissues for stability, having no prosthetic hinge.

The main advantage of these implants is the significantly reduced stress transmission at the bone–cement and cement–prosthesis interfaces. Forces are absorbed by the soft tissues (capsule, ligaments, and muscles) surrounding the prosthesis, leading to better preservation of bone stock, decreased polyethylene wear, and preservation of normal elbow kinematics, ultimately decreasing the risk of implant loosening. However, imperfect balance and component maltracking due to uncorrected angulation or rotation can lead to asymmetric polyethylene loading, a decreased joint surface contact area, and increased wear [4]. Of course, such imbalance can also predispose the joint to instability. The main drawback of this implant is that it requires good articular balance, with an intact capsule and collateral ligaments. The rarity of this condition in patients requiring elbow replacement limits the indications for these implants.

The majority of unlinked TEAs lack a radial head prosthesis, with only a few designs allowing its substitution. Although, in theory, the radial head component improves soft tissue balance and has been shown to enhance stability in in-vitro biomechanical studies [5], in vivo results for TEAs using prostheses with radial head components have been disappointing. The radial head prosthesis in the original capital–condylar total elbow prosthesis was usually abandoned because it was considered to contribute to the loosening of the humeral component, delivering asymmetrical stress forces across the elbow [5].

Convertible prosthesis: With these designs, it is possible to convert intraoperatively or in further surgeries from a hemiarthroplasty or an unlinked implant to a linked elbow arthroplasty, depending to the condition of the patient's elbow [6]. The conversion from one design to another can be performed without removing stable components, but only by modifying the linking mechanism [7].

Due to their ability to guarantee joint stability, linked implants are indicated in cases of severe bone loss and joint instability, such as complex comminuted fractures, severe osteoarthritis with joint disruption, osteonecrosis, hemophilic arthropathy, and rheumatoid arthritis.

6.3 Planning

In prosthetic arthroplasty, proper implant placement is essential to reducing the incidence of complications. However, unlike planning for knee and hip replacement, for which many reports have demonstrated the usefulness of three-dimensional (3D) templates based on computed tomography (CT), only a limited number of studies have described prosthetic arthroplasty of the upper limb, with sporadic reports on total shoulder arthroplasty. Iwamoto et al. designed a study based on the planning of 39 patients undergoing unlinked total elbow replacement. This system generates reconstructed images in three orthogonal planes, facilitating the measurement of angles and distances between any two points in each plane. Measurements are performed using four-point method for the humerus and six-point method for the ulna [8].

6.4 Surgical Approach of TEA

When planning an elbow arthroplasty, some key factors have to be kept in consideration, in particular bone stock, ligamentous stability, and triceps integrity.

- **Bone stock** is represented by the distal humerus, ulna, and radial head.
- When planning the prosthetic implant and selecting the optimal surgical approach, the surgeon must assess the extent of distal humerus involvement due to the lesion, fracture, or degenerative process. In case of massive and more proximal humeral damage, a long stem implant must be available, along with solutions for bone stock deficit (bone grafting, cerclages, and so on). The radial head, when present, is usually resected and in some cases, a radial head implant is part of the total elbow replacement (especially in unlinked designs).
- Ulnar bone stock has primary importance in elbow replacement: to properly position the ulnar component, no fractures should be present, if present, they must be carefully considered because of the extreme complexity of their intraoperative management while performing a total elbow replacement. For this reason, in cases of comminuted distal humerus fractures, if in doubt between ORIF and replacement, it is strongly advised to avoid performing an olecranon osteotomy. This procedure will significantly increases the complexity of elbow replacement, so if in doubt, an alternative approach [9].
- **Ligaments** must be assessed preoperatively: In cases of comminuted distal humerus fractures, ligament evaluation is not feasible, leading directly to the

choide of a linked implant. Otherwise, in degenerative joint disease, a well-preserved ligamentous complex may allow for the use of an unlinked prosthesis or, at least, a convertible implant.
- **The triceps** serve as the "engine" of an elbow replacement, and preserving the integrity of the extensor apparatus is crucial. The management of the triceps tendon in the surgical approach to elbow replacement is a key factor, and must be considered [10–12].

6.5 Surgical Procedure

A posterior longitudinal incision is typically used, with a lateral or medial curve around the tip of the olecranon process to achieve optimal visualization of both the medial and lateral compartments. Before exposing the joint, the ulnar nerve must be identified and carefully mobilized to prevent injury, ensuring it is safely retracted away from the surgical field [1].

6.6 Triceps Approaches

There are three main modalities of approaching the triceps: reflecting, splitting, and preserving. The choice depends on the surgeon's preference and the elbow conditions. When possible, preserving the triceps is crucial, as its integrity is essential to achieve early mobilization and prevent complications such as local pain, weakness, and stiffness.

The triceps reflecting procedure was proposed by Bryan-Morrey in 1982. The triceps is medially isolated and progressively detached from the olecranon insertion, reflecting the tendon itself laterally, preserving its distal ulnar insertion. In this process, detaching a bony fragment from the tip of the olecranon can be useful for optimizing tendon tension during reinsertion at the end of the procedure.

The main advantage of this procedure is the good vision and easy approach to both the humerus and the ulna. As a drawback, the tendon is almost completely detached from the ulna, requiring time for healing, and triceps weakness is sometimes observed [12–14].

The triceps splitting procedure is similar, but the triceps is split in the midline all the way on to the olecranon, preserving only the distal insertion (Fig. 6.1). The tendon is then detached from the olecranon and reflected both laterally and medially from the midline, allowing the surgeon to place the implant via the split [15, 16].

As for the triceps reflecting approach, the main advantages are the good joint exposure and the low complexity, but as drawbacks, the extensor apparatus is weakened and may not heal properly. As in the reflecting approach, the rehabilitation should be careful, and a postoperative boutonniere deformity of the triceps may be observed due to the nonhealing and shortening of the detached component [16].

A triceps preserving procedure is performed when the surgeon aims to avoid triceps weakening. The triceps is isolated both medially and laterally, usually with

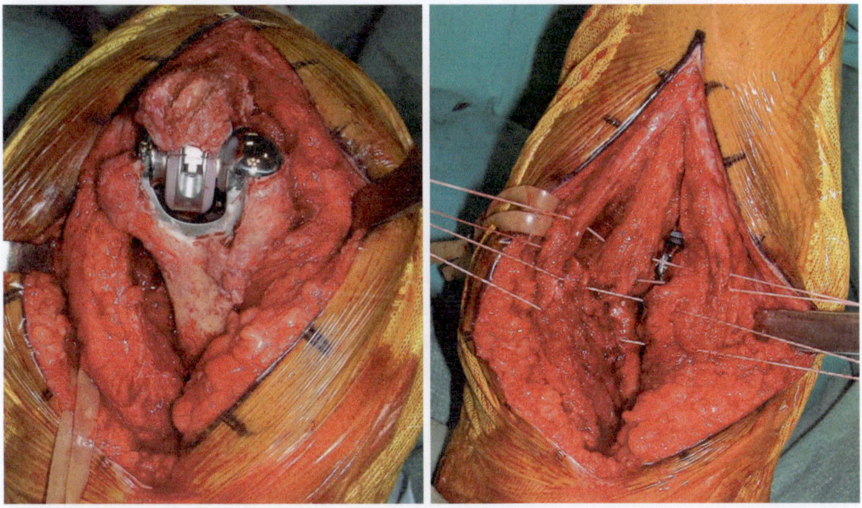

Fig. 6.1 Triceps splitting approach

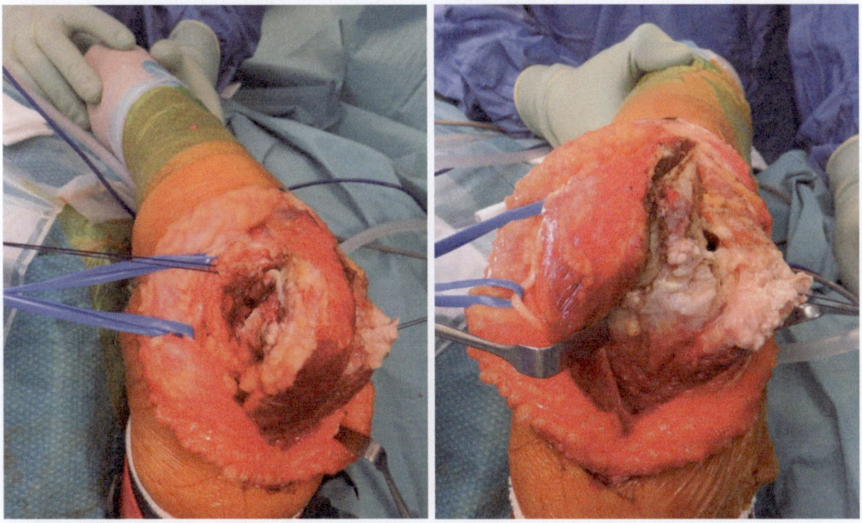

Fig. 6.2 Para-olecranon approach, both medial and lateral view, described by King [18]

a paraolecranon approach that exposes the lateral and medial aspects of the olecranon. This allows access to and preparation of the joint from both sides of the triceps, while preserving its insertion on the olecranon process [17, 18] (Fig. 6.2).

This approach is ideal for preserving the triceps, allowing an early rehabilitation and active movement also in elbow extension. In addition, it is easier to achieve good joint tension, avoiding elongation or shortening of the joint, using the triceps tension as a landmark for component insertion. On the other hand, ulnar preparation is more challenging because of the limited exposure and the bulkiness of the triceps tendon, making component reduction more complex.

In selected cases of prosthesis revision or hemiarthroplasty, the TRAP (triceps reflecting anconeus pedicle) approach can be useful: the triceps is reflected proximally, maintaining its continuity with the anconeus muscle, which is also isolated, detached, and proximally reflected (Fig. 6.3).

This approach allows a wide joint view but requires a big exposure with soft tissue detaching and may cause triceps weakening and a delay in physiotherapy.

Once the surgical approach with optimal triceps management has been planned, the implant is placed following the standard technique.

It is important to perform a good capsulotomy and ligament release to obtain an optimal joint view. A key aspect of the surgery is the identification of the flexion–extension axis of the elbow [19]. This axis can be identified by drawing a virtual line from the ligamentous insertion of the LCL on the lateral epicondyle to the insertion point of the MCL, located anterior and inferior to the medial epicondyle. However, in some cases, particularly in distal humerus fractures, it can be difficult to identify the flexion–extension axis [20] (Fig. 6.4).

When these anatomic landmarks are not identifiable, it is important to consider that lengthening the humeral component an result in flexion contracture and limited elbow extension. For this reason, it is preferable to position the implant slightly

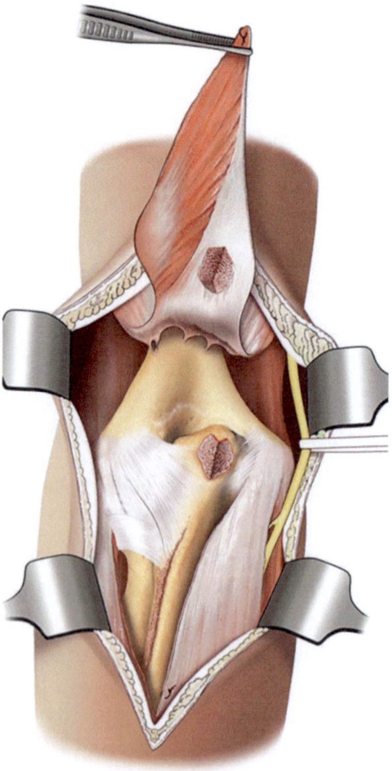

Fig. 6.3 TRAP approach.

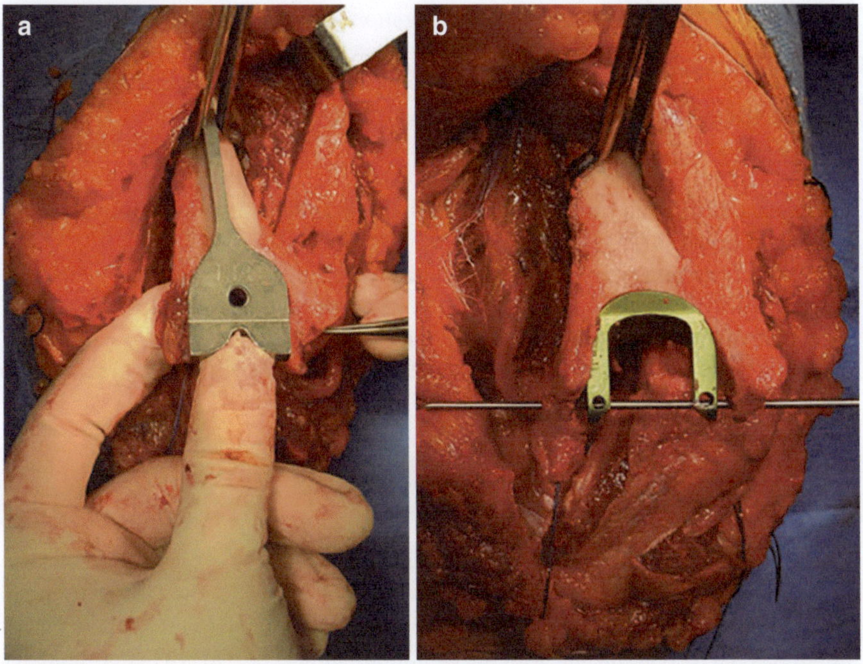

Fig. 6.4 (**a**) Visualization of the flexion–extension axis between the epicondyles. (**b**) Visualization of the height of the F–E axis to perform trial implant. Reproduced with permission from "Scacchi, M., Giannicola, G. (2020). Indications and Surgical Technique of Primary Elbow Linked Arthroplasty. In: Castoldi, F., Giannicola, G., Rotini, R. (eds) Elbow Arthroplasty. Springer, Cham." https://doi.org/10.1007/978-3-030-14455-5_6

shorter [21]. When the distal humerus is preserved and the rotation axis is identifiable, the surgeon can accurately perform the humeral cut and correctly place the prosthesis, starting with the identification of the medullary canal using a high-speed burr to perforate the posterior cortex that limits the superior part of the olecranon fossa. During this procedure, it is essential to pay attention in patients with osteoporotic bones or in case of post-traumatic deformities to avoid intraoperative fracture. Attention is also required to avoid implant malposition in varus–valgus angulation on the frontal plane or flexion–extension on the sagittal plane. For this reason, preoperative planning with a CT scan is mandatory. Once the humeral canal has been prepared, the humeral component can be trial-fitted to verify the correct orientation and size. During this phase, it is important to evaluate the right rotation of the implant, considering that the posterior cortex is externally rotated by 14.0° ± 4.2° in the F–E axis and this rotation is slightly smaller in males than in females [22]. The implant is then positioned with its posterior aspect in line with the posterior cortex and rotated internally by 15°. Another method to evaluate the correct position of the trial humeral component is by using the trans-epicondylar axis, which is determined by drawing a line between the most prominent points on the epicondyles. This line then tipically requires an external rotation of a mean of 2.8° ± 3.5° relative to the F–E axis [22]. Once the humeral preparation is complete, the ulna is prepared, starting with an accurate removal of osteophytes followed by preparation of the ulnar canal. The goal in this final phase is to place the ulnar component in a position that reproduces the natural center of rotation of the greater sigmoid notch [22, 23].

In this phase, it is necessary to pay attention to the following three aspects:

- The axis of rotation should lie approximately equidistant between the olecranon and coronoid tip [23] [24].
- The articular portion of the ulnar implant must run perpendicular between two landmarks: the ulnar crest of the sigmoid notch and the so-called "flat zone," located in the flat posterior portion of the olecranon.
- Obtain an adequate anterior–posterior offset, which refers to a virtual center of a circle inscribed into the greater sigmoid notch [24].

Osteophytosis of the coronoid tip must be removed before the ulnar component implantation to avoid the "pistoning effect" against the humerus during maximum flexion.

With a linked implant, the radial head can be left, excised, or replaced. It is usually left in situ because the native radial head can be used as a graft for an eventual revision. If the choice is to cut the radial head, it is preferable to do so at the end of the surgery, as its relationship with the capitulum humeri provides a better reference for evaluating the implant positioning. The final evaluation must focus on the balance and tension of the triceps. This maneuver, called the "shuck test," consists of flexing the forearm to 90° and then pulling it away from the humerus as much as the soft tissues allow. At this stage, the importance of preserving the tricipital insertion during the approach becomes apparent [24, 25] (Fig. 6.5).

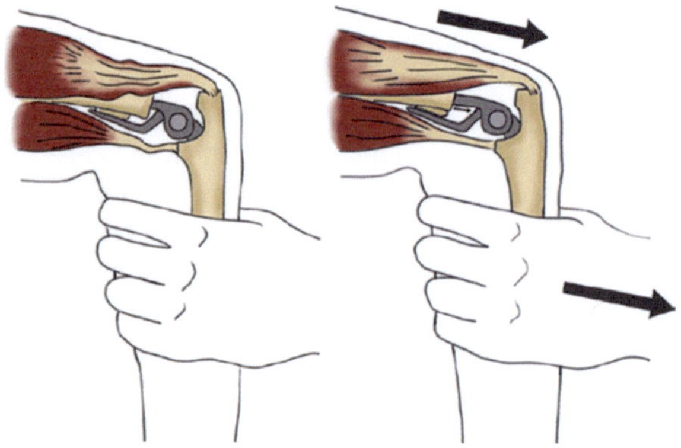

Fig. 6.5 Shuck test. Reproduced with permission from "Scacchi, M., Giannicola, G. (2020). Indications and Surgical Technique of Primary Elbow Linked Arthroplasty. In: Castoldi, F., Giannicola, G., Rotini, R. (eds) Elbow Arthroplasty. Springer, Cham." https://doi.org/10.1007/978-3-030-14455-5_6

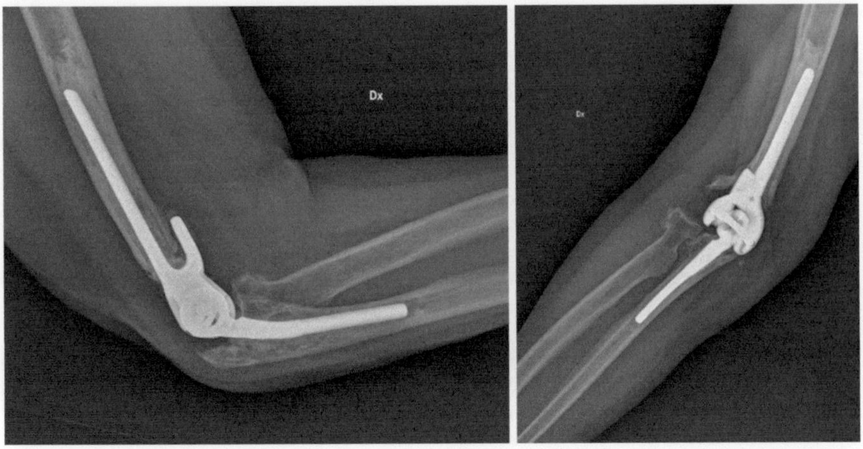

Fig. 6.6 Final X-ray of a TEA

The final step of the surgery is the cementation of the implant. Adequate cementation is fundamental for the survivorship of the implant. Two-stage cementation may help prevent some intraoperative and early complications such as fractures and malpositioning [24, 26]. If linked implants are used, the surgeon may choose whether to repair or not the collateral ligaments (Fig. 6.6).

Take Home Messages

1. TEA is a procedure with several limitations for the patient. Its surgical indications are very restricted compared to other prostheses.
2. Semi-constrained or linked implant designs are the most commonly available and used on the market.
3. Bone stock, ligamentous stability, and triceps conditions are the most important parameters that need to be evaluated when performing a TEA.
4. For a good implant placement, the rotational axis and the articular surface of the ulnar component need to be used as reference parameters.

References

1. Day JS, Lau E, Ong KL, Williams GR, Ramsey ML, Kurtz SM. Prevalence and projections of total shoulder and elbow arthroplasty in the United States to 2015. Shoulder Elbow Surg. 2010;19(8):1115–20. https://doi.org/10.1016/j.jse.2010.02.009.
2. Gay DM, Lyman S, Do H, Hotchkiss RN, Marx RG, Daluisk A. Indications and reoperation rates for total elbow arthroplasty: an analysis of trends in New York State. J Bone Joint Surg Am. 2012;94(2):1107. https://doi.org/10.2106/JBJS.J.01128.
3. Celli A, Morrey BF. Total elbow arthroplasty in patients forty years of age or less. J Bone Joint Surg Am. 2009;91(6):1414–8. https://doi.org/10.2106/JBJS.G.00329.

4. Plaschke HC, Thillemann TM, Brorson S, Olsen BS. Implant survival after total elbow arthroplasty: a retrospective study of 324 procedures performed from 1980 to 2008. J Shoulder Elb Surg. 2014;23:829–36. https://doi.org/10.1016/j.jse.2014.02.001.
5. Ewald FC, Scheinberg RD, Poss R, Thomas WH, Scott RD, Sledge CB. Capitellocondylar total elbow arthroplasty. J Bone Joint Surg Am. 1980;62:1259–63.
6. Kamineni S, O'Driscoll SW, Urban M, Garg A, Berglund LJ, Morrey BF, An KN. Intrinsic constraint of unlinked total elbow replacements--the ulnotrochlear joint. J Bone Joint Surg Am. 2005;87(9):2019–27. https://doi.org/10.2106/JBJS.C.00983.
7. Chafik D, O'Driscoll S, King GW, Yamaguchi K. Total elbow arthroplasty-convertible. Oper Techn Orthop. 2010;20(1):58–67.
8. Iwamoto T, Suzuki T, Oki S, Matsumura N, Nakamura M, Matsumoto M, Sato K. Computed tomography-based 3-dimensional pre-operative planning for unlinked total elbow arthroplasty. J Shoulder Elb Surg. 2018;27(10):1792–9. https://doi.org/10.1016/j.jse.2018.04.013.
9. Morrey ME, Morrey BF, Sanchez-Sotelo J, Barlow JD, O'Driscoll S. A review of the surgical management of distal humerus fractures and nonunions: from fixation to arthroplasty. J Clin Orthop Trauma. 2021;20:101477. https://doi.org/10.1016/j.jcot.2021.101477.
10. Sanchez-Sotelo J. Total elbow arthroplasty. Open Orthop J. 2011;5:115–23. https://doi.org/10.2174/1874325001105010115.
11. Celli A, Arash A, Adams RA, Morrey BF. Triceps insufficiency following total elbow arthroplasty. J Bone Joint Surg Am. 2005;87(9):1957–64. https://doi.org/10.2106/JBJS.D.02423.
12. Morrey BF, Sanchez-Sotelo J. Approaches for elbow arthroplasty: how to handle the triceps. J Shoulder Elb Surg. 2011;20(2 Suppl):S90–6. https://doi.org/10.1016/j.jse.2010.12.004.
13. Poon PC, Foliaki S, Young SW, Eisenhauer D. Triceps Split and Snip approach to the elbow: surgical technique and biomechanical evaluation. ANZ J Surg. 2013;83(10):774–8. https://doi.org/10.1111/ans.12131.
14. Celli A. A new posterior triceps approach for total elbow arthroplasty in patients with osteoarthritis secondary to fracture: preliminary clinical experience. J Shoulder Elb Surg. 2016;25(8):e223–31. https://doi.org/10.1016/j.jse.2016.04.003.
15. Campbell WC. Campbell's operative orthopedics. St. Louis: MO Mosby; 1971. p. 119J.
16. Campbell WC. Incision for exposure of the elbow joint. Am J Surg. 1932;15:65–7. https://doi.org/10.1016/S0002-9610(32)90997-0.
17. Alonso-Llames M. Bilaterotricipital approach to the elbow. Acta Orthop Scand. 1972;43(6):479–90. https://doi.org/10.3109/17453677208991270.
18. Studer A, Athwal GS, MacDermid JC, Faber KJ, King GJW. The lateral para-olecranon approach for total elbow arthroplasty. J Hand Surg Am. 2013;38(11):2219–2226.e3. https://doi.org/10.1016/j.jhsa.2013.07.029.
19. Brownhill JR, Furukawa K, Faber KJ, Johnson JA, King GJW. Surgeon accuracy in the selection of the flexion-extension axis of the elbow: an in vitro study. J Shoulder Elb Surg. 2006;15(4):451–6. https://doi.org/10.1016/j.jse.2005.09.011.
20. Lenoir H, Chammas M, Micallef JP, Lazerges C, Waitzenegger T, Coulet B. The effect of the anatomy of the distal humerus and proximal ulna on the positioning of the components in total elbow arthroplasty. Bone Joint J. 2015;97-B(11):1539–45. https://doi.org/10.1302/0301-620X.97B11.36071.
21. Donald H. Lee. Linked total elbow arthroplasty. Hand Clin. 2011;27(2):199–213., vi. https://doi.org/10.1016/j.hcl.2011.01.004.
22. Sabo MT, Athwal GS, King GJW. Landmarks for rotational alignment of the humeral component during elbow arthroplasty. J Bone Joint Surg Am. 2012;94(19):1794–800. https://doi.org/10.2106/JBJS.J.01740.
23. Kamineni S. Distal humerus fractures. In: Morrey BF, Sanchez-Sotelo J, Morrey M, editors. The elbow and its disorders. 5th ed. Elsevier; 2018. p. 878–87.
24. Sacchi M, Giannicola G. Chapter 6: Indication and surgical technique of primary elbow linked arthroplasty. In: Castoldi F, Giannicola G, Rotini R, editors. Elbow arthroplasty: current techniques and complications. Springer Nature; 2020. p. 77–96.

25. Sánchez-Sotelo J, Morrey B. Linked elbow replacement: a salvage procedure for distal humeral nonunion. Surgical technique. J Bone Joint Surg Am. 2009;91(Suppl 2):200–12. https://doi.org/10.2106/JBJS.I.00383.
26. Giannicola G, Scacchi M, Polimanti D, Cinotti G. Discovery elbow system: 2- to 5-year results in distal humerus fractures and post-traumatic conditions: a prospective study on 24 patients. J Hand Surg Am. 2014;39(9):1746–56. https://doi.org/10.1016/j.jhsa.2014.05.027.

Planning in Elbow Hemiarthroplasty

7

C. Buondonno, A. Marinelli, L. Ferra, M. Riva, A. Sessa, and E. Guerra

7.1 Introduction

Elbow hemiarthroplasty (EHA) consists of the partial replacement of the elbow joint, involving only the humeral component. It is composed of three modular parts: (1) a stem that needs to be cemented; (2) an anatomical spool designed to replicate the distal humerus shape; (3) a cannulated pin, which is used to connect the spool to the stem (Fig. 7.1).

Over the last decade, EHA has become, especially in Europe, a promising treatment option for elbow joint diseases that affect the distal humerus, including fractures, nonunions, intrinsic post-traumatic stiffness, and avascular necrosis [1–8].

EHA tries to overcome the current limits of open reduction and internal fixation (ORIF) and of total elbow arthroplasty (TEA).

ORIF is still considered the gold standard for distal humeral fractures. However, despite the improvement in internal fixation technique, there remains a subset of fractures (usually B3, A2.3, and C according to AO classification) that are difficult to reconstruct for their poor bone quality and articular comminution. In these cases, ORIF should not be sought at any cost, especially in elderly patients, and elbow replacement is indicated.

TEA has proved to be a satisfying treatment option in elderly patients, but complication rates are still higher than in other joints. In particular, TEA may lead to early loosening, necessitating revision, especially in high-demand patients. The theoretical advantages of EHA over TEA are the absence of polyethylene debris with the consequent osteolysis and the less weight restrictions, especially in younger and still active patients. As the ulnar component has the highest risk of loosening, using an EHA eliminate this risk, but complications such as periprosthetic fracture

C. Buondonno · A. Marinelli · L. Ferra · M. Riva · A. Sessa · E. Guerra (✉)
Shoulder and Elbow Unit – IRCCS, Istituto Ortopedico Rizzoli, Bologna, Italy
e-mail: enrico.guerra@ior.it

G. M. Marcheggiani Muccioli et al. (eds.), *Easy Planning in Elective Primary Orthopedic Procedures*, https://doi.org/10.1007/978-3-031-77006-7_7

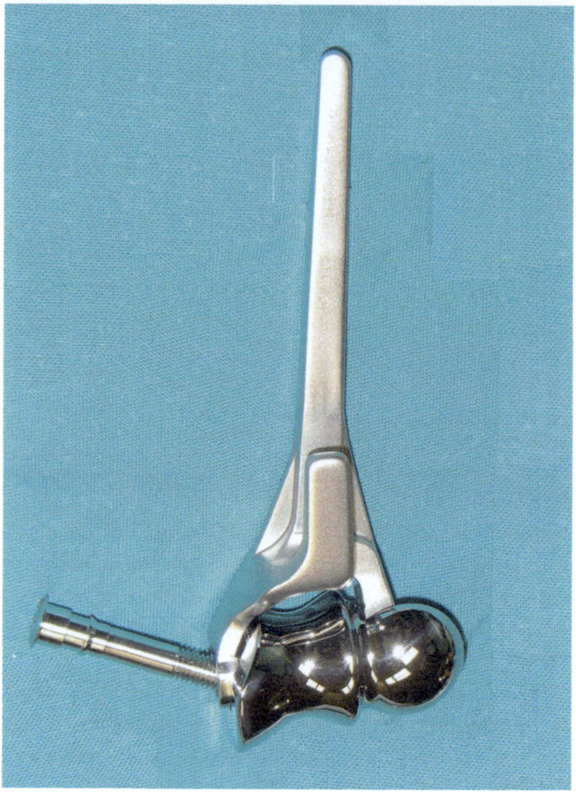

Fig. 7.1 EHA is composed of a flanged stem, an anatomical spool, and a cannulated pin that connects the previous two parts

and PMMMA wear may still occur. Compared to TEA, the potential disadvantages are the risk of instability, with progressive joint osteoarthritis due to the direct contact of the metallic trochlea against the articular surfaces of the greater sigmoid notch and radial head.

7.2 Indications

Unreconstructable acute fractures of the distal humerus represent the primary surgical indication of EHA. Other possible indications for EHA are as salvage of post-traumatic sequelae related to nonoperative management or failed articular humeral fixation (nonunion, malunion, intrinsic stiffness), as well as in other rare pathological conditions as distal humerus avascular necrosis or tumors not involving the humeral columns [7, 9].

EHA implants are inherently unconstrained, so joint stability relies on the congruence of their design with the radioulnar surfaces and on the integrity or stable reconstruction of the primary and secondary elbow stabilizers: medial and lateral columns with their corresponding collateral ligaments, radial head, olecranon, and coronoid [7].

Should the need for TEA revision arise, the current prosthetic system allows the conversion from EHA to TEA (unlinked or linked) without humeral component removal.

7.3 Contraindications

Absolute contraindications are represented by contaminated open fractures or chronic infection of the elbow. EHA is also contraindicated in case of not fixable medial or lateral columns, irreparable MCL (Medial Collateral Ligament) or LCL (Lateral Collateral Ligament), lesions or fractures of the radial head, coronoid, or olecranon that cannot be stably fixed. In those cases, a linked TEA should be considered. Relative contraindications to EHA are preexisting degenerative ulnar osteoarthritis due to the risk of persistence or increase of *postoperative pain* and stiffness. Contraindications to EHA also include younger patients with complex but fixable fractures [1, 7].

7.4 Preoperative Planning

Before considering performing an EHA, careful and accurate planning is necessary [10].

Medical History The presence of concomitant diseases, level of physical activity, and needs of the patient must be evaluated. Metal hypersensitivity and previous surgeries around the elbow must be investigated, and the attesting documents and surgical reports must be asked for.

Clinical Evaluation The elbow skin condition must be checked and the presence of previous scars, an open fracture, or an ongoing local infection must be ruled out. The neurovascular condition of the involved upper limb must be examined; in particular, the ulnar nerve condition must be addressed, reporting any weakness or numbness. The position of the ulnar nerve must be assessed to evaluate if a previous transposition has been performed.

Imaging Imaging evaluation must confirm the not-fixable involvement of the distal humerus while assessing the integrity or repairability of the bony and soft tissue stabilizers. Orthogonal plain radiographs are almost always completed by computed tomography (CT) with 2D and 3D reconstruction. Unfortunately, virtual planning software allowing to plan or navigate the surgery are not available for elbow replacement at the moment.

Instrumentation The surgeon must ensure that the necessary instrumentation to implant the humeral prosthesis and to repair the elbow stabilizers if they are injured is available. To date, Latitude EV implant (Tornier, Wright Medical, Texas) is the only hemiarthroplasty implant available on the market (Fig. 7.2).

It is an anatomic, modular, and cemented implant with an interchangeable spool for conversion to linked or unlinked TEA, without the need for humeral exchange. The spool is cannulated to allow ligament repair through the center of rotation of the implant.

In addition to the elbow replacement system provided by the company, other necessary instruments to have in the operating room are tourniquet, bean bag if the lateral decubitus is decided, oscillating saw, high-speed burr, low-viscosity cement, cement restrictor and gun, and C-arm machine for intraoperative fluoroscopy (Fig. 7.3).

Moreover, anatomical distal humerus plates, Kirschner wires, cannulated washer screws, anchors, and high-strength sutures are the devices most commonly used to reconstruct or repair elbow stabilizers.

In case of previous failed osteosynthesis, a detailed list of the previously implanted hardware is needed to allow the surgeon to prepare the specific removal tools. The previous operative report is useful in understanding the triceps management formerly performed and confirming the ulnar nerve position.

It is always necessary to have the necessary instruments available for conversion to a total prosthesis, even when the initial plan is to perform a partial prosthesis. Sometimes, is not possible to implanting a partial prosthesis. This may occur in

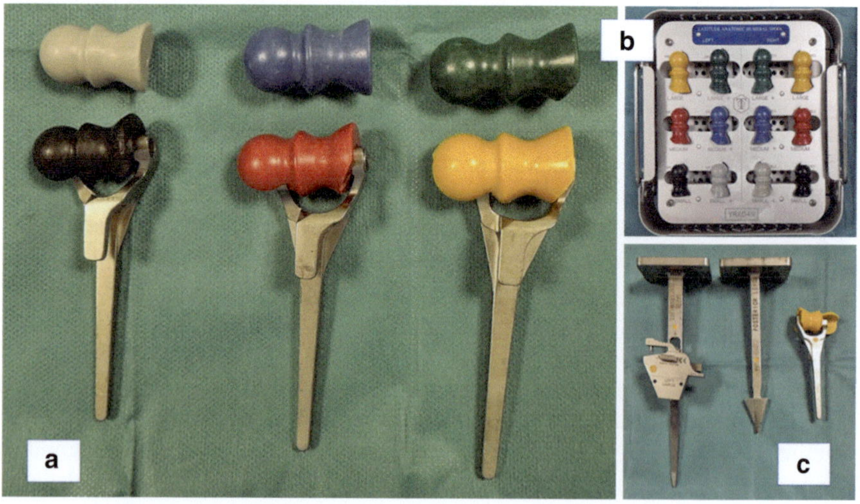

Fig. 7.2 Latitude EV trial instrumentation. (**a**) Anatomic humeral stems are of three different sizes (small black, medium red, large yellow). (**b**) Anatomic spools are of six different sizes for right and six for left side (small black, small + gray, medium red, medium + blue, large yellow, large + green). (**c**) Humeral broaches and humeral cut guides are specific for each trial stem

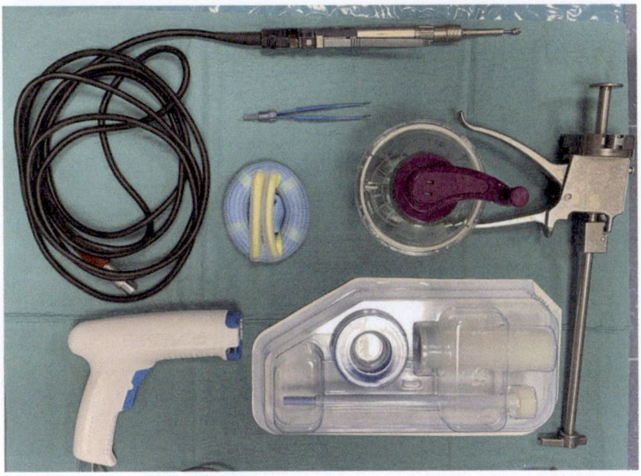

Fig. 7.3 Some of the needed instrumentations are depicted (sterile tourniquet, high-speed burr, bipolar forceps, tools for preparing the cementation)

cases of intraoperative evidence of ulnar arthritis not shown by instrumental examinations before, mismatch between the spool and the large sigmoid notch given the few available measurements, irreparability of the columns or of the ligaments, and the presence of residual instability.

Informed Consent EHA is a complex operation, potentially even more difficult than ORIF and TEA if performed by inexperienced surgeons. Because of the possible alternative treatments and complications, exhaustive informed consent is necessary before performing EHA. Providing the patient with detailed information about his/her current elbow condition, and the available solutions, and informing about realistic expectations and possible complications of an elbow replacement fosters trust in the patient–physician relationship and allows the patient to take part in the decision-making process.

7.5 Surgical Approach Decision

The strategic choice of surgical exposure is certainly the first basic step to obtaining a good EHA implant and minimizing complications. EHA can be implanted using several approaches, each with its advantages and limits. Regardless of the selected approach, the insertion of the elbow prosthesis requires the management of the elbow extensor mechanism to expose the joint, to reach space for joint resection, to determine the correct insertion and size of the implant, and to handle collateral ligaments and condyles. Whenever it is possible, preserving the triceps attachment reduces the risk of overstuffing and of extensor system weakness, allowing early active motion in the postoperative phase.

Based on the different triceps management, the most suggested approaches to implant an EHA can be divided into five groups:

1. Approaches sparing all the olecranon triceps insertion:

Triceps-on [3].
Kocher extensile [11].
Medial epicondyle osteotomy [12]/medial opening through the epitrochlear fracture

2. Approaches sparing a good portion of the olecranon triceps insertion:
   Lateral para-olecranon approach [10, 13].
3. Approaches detaching all the triceps insertion from the olecranon:
   Triceps splitting (Campbell) [5].
   Triceps-reflecting anconeus pedicle (TRAP) [14].
   Adolfsson–Nestorson modified splitting approach [8].
4. Approaches detaching the olecranon through an osteotomy:
   Olecranon osteotomy [15, 16].
5. Approaches splitting the triceps at the musculotendinous interface:
   Tongue approach [17, 18].

The choice among these approaches should be based on the specific elbow disorders, such as the concomitant acute column fractures or the presence of associated fractures (olecranon, for example), of hardware and considering the specific surgeon preferences.

- **Triceps-on:**

This approach has been ideated in order to preserve the whole triceps insertion that remains attached to the olecranon. Nowadays, this is the most suggested approach to implant EHA in acute C2 and C3 AO classification distal humeral fractures (Fig. 7.4) [7, 11]. The distal humerus is exposed through a medial and lateral window, moving the triceps from one side to another of the humerus. In EHA implants, this approach is particularly indicated when the distal humerus fracture is associated with a fracture involving both columns. The column fractures, with their preserved collateral ligaments, are retracted to expose the distal humerus and then, after EHA implantation, they are reduced and fixed by plates, screws, K wires, or bony sutures based on their size and comminution. This approach, sparing all the triceps insertion, facilitates an early unrestricted range of motion and prevents the risk of triceps failure.

- **Kocher extensile:**

This approach allows the exposure of the anterior and posterior part of the capitulum and the anterior part of the trochlea through a dislocating maneuver using the intact medial column and medial collateral as a hinge. It is indicated in comminuted capitellar–trochlear shear fractures that are unfixable [11]. If the lateral column is fractured, it can be exploited to subluxate the ulnohumeral joint without detaching the lateral collateral ligament. The exposure consists proximally in a lateral column procedure with release of the triceps from the posterior column of the common extensor tendons and capsule from their humeral insertion. The lateral column fracture with the inserted LCL is carefully retracted. Distally, the approach is extended

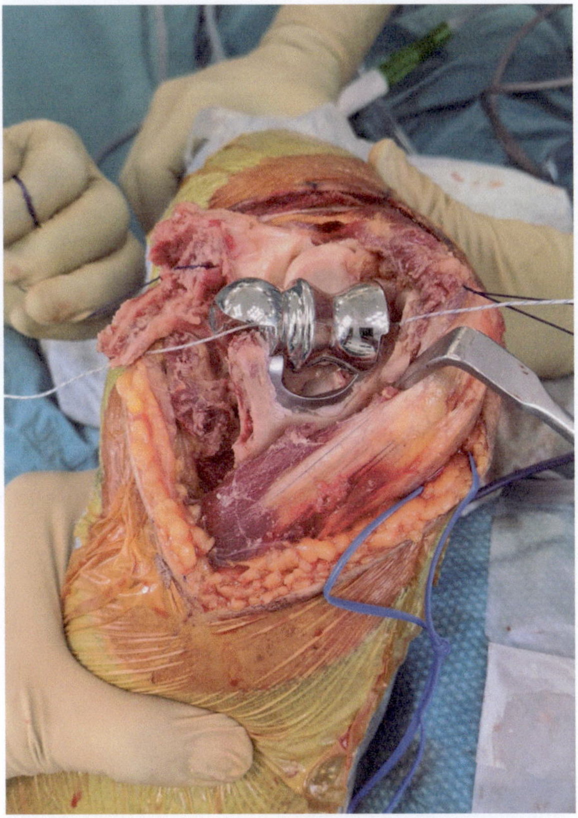

Fig. 7.4 Triceps on approach allows for good intra-articular view, especially in case of column fractures as shown in this case. The triceps insertion is preserved so that the triceps tension can be used as an important landmark to identify the correct length of the implant. With this approach, an unrestricted range of motion can be allowed to the patient in the early postoperative phase

in the Kocher interval between anconeus, which is partially detached from its ulnar insertion and extensor carpi ulnaris. Applying a varus, flexion, and supination force, a subluxation maneuver is achieved, using the MCL and common flexor muscles as a hinge to dislocate the elbow. This approach allows a wide exposure of the articular anterior surface of the distal humerus. After the EHA has been implanted, the lateral column is usually fixed with an anatomical plate.

- **Medial approach through epitrochlear fracture:**

The approach through the medial condyle can be used to implant an EHA in case of not-fixable distal humerus articular fractures associated with a fracture of the medial column [12]. In these cases, it is possible to take advantage of the medial column fracture and dislocate the elbow through a valgus and pronation maneuver, pivoting the joint on an intact lateral column and lateral ulnar collateral ligament (LUCL). This approach allows a wide exposure to the joint. Once EHA has been implanted, the medial column is fixed, usually with an anatomical plate or cannulated screws.

- **Para-olecranon:**

The lateral para-olecranon approach exposed the ulnohumeral joint through medial and lateral arthrotomies, leaving the insertion of the central triceps tendon attached to the olecranon [13]. The posterolateral arthrotomy is performed distally to the olecranon using the Boyd approach. Proximally, the triceps tendon is split between the central tendinous attachment to the olecranon and its lateral expansion and the lateral half of the triceps. The lateral part of the triceps, along with the anconeus, is retracted laterally as a single unit. If a lateral column fragment, including the common extensor tendon and lateral ulnar collateral ligament, is present, they do not have to be released. On the medial side, the ulnar nerve is released and transposed, the triceps muscle is released from the medial intermuscular septum and dorsal aspect of the distal humerus. If a medial column fragment, including the common flexor tendon and the medial ulnar collateral ligament, is present, they do not have to be elevated off the medial epicondyle. The fractured articular fragments are removed to gain access to the distal humerus, taking care to spare the epicondyles with their attached collateral ligaments. At the end of the surgery, if the humeral columns are fractured, they are fixed to the humeral component [10], if the humeral columns are intact, the medial and lateral soft tissues are repaired back to the distal humerus. The triceps split is then closed. This approach allows immediate triceps use without risk of triceps failure.

- **Triceps splitting:**

This approach, initially described by Campbell, which consists in dissecting longitudinally the triceps, detaching its insertion on both sides of the olecranon, is particularly indicated in cases where there are no column fractures. Using this approach, to dislocate the elbow, it is necessary to release the collateral ligaments from the condyles. At the end of surgery, after having implanted the prosthesis, the ligaments must be sutured to the bone and the two sides of this soft tissue "envelope" must be closed using side-to-side stiches. The triceps needs to be reattached to the olecranon as strongly as possible with multiple trans-osseous sutures. Shahane-Stanley [19] proposed a modification of this technique, performing the triceps split 75% laterally and 25% medially. The medial part is then detached subperiosteally and reflected medially as a single unit, the lateral part of the triceps with the anconeus, and the extensors are dissected according to the needs of the procedure being undertaken. Lately, Nestorson et al. [8] described in a small number of cases of EHA implantation, a modification of the original Campbell approach with a mid-line triceps split and detaching only the lateral half of the triceps and leaving the medial half inserted on the olecranon. Through this approach, the joint can be dislocated, and the humeral canal can be prepared. More recently, Phadnis et al. [3] published a case series where the triceps had been split in lateral one-third and medial two-thirds with a second window performed on the medial border of the triceps to access the medial condyle and collateral ligament.

- **Triceps-reflecting anconeus pedicle (TRAP):**

This approach consists of detaching the triceps-anconeus unit from its ulnar and humeral insertion to expose the distal humerus [14]. This exposure has the advantage of allowing a wide exposure of the distal humerus without performing an olecranon osteotomy. The approach is particularly indicated when the decision to proceed with internal fixation or arthroplasty (EHA or TEA) needs to be taken intraoperatively. The advantage of this approach is that it allows a wide access to the joint, avoiding the olecranon osteotomy, but it has the disadvantage that it can cause a triceps weakness.

- **Olecranon osteotomy:**

This approach allows the greatest joint exposure. It is exploited when the surgeon wishes to maximize the ORIF's chances of success in a comminuted articular fracture of the distal humerus. This approach is, therefore, particularly indicated in young or relatively young patients, where the EHA replacement is not desired, and it is considered only as a salvage procedure if, despite all attempts, the fixation is impossible to obtain. Using the olecranon osteotomy approach, it is, in fact, possible the intra-operative conversion from ORIF to EHA but, in case of an unexpected instability with the necessity to consider a TEA, surgical difficulties grow much more. This approach is associated with possible complications such as osteotomy delayed union, nonunion, malunion, prominent hardware, intra-articular adhesions, and arthritis. Moreover, the intact sigmoid notch is important in choosing the implant spool size, and the triceps tension is an important landmark in identifying the correct length of the implant: for all these reasons, the olecranon osteotomy is not the ideal approach to performing an EHA.

- **Tongue approach:**

The triceps fascial tongue approach, originally described in 1940 by Van Gorder for T-type distal humeral fractures, has been recently proposed as a possible approach for intra-articular distal humeral fracture fixation [20, 21] and total elbow arthroplasty [17, 18]. Although to date the tongue approach has never been described to implant an EHA, it should be considered as a possible approach. Especially, after having dissected the collateral ligament from the ulnar insertion, and proposed by O'Driscoll in 2018, it provides adequate visualization of the articular surface, allowing an easy conversion from ORIF to EHA or TEA if necessary.

Take Home Messages

1. Elbow hemiarthroplasty is indicated in selected patients with acute traumatic injuries, in some of their sequelae or, rarely, in other elbow disorders, as avascular necrosis or tumors.

2. The recent literature shows a growing number of case series reporting a high rate of satisfactory results and long survival rates at short- to medium-term follow-ups [1–6, 8, 9, 16, 22, 23].
3. The surgical technique to implant an EHA is complex and that the potential complications are numerous and not always easy to solve.
4. To maximize the results and to limit the complications, surgical planning must be performed with careful attention.

References

1. Phadnis J, Watts AC, Bain GI. Elbow hemiarthroplasty for the management of distal humeral fractures: current technique, indications and results. Shoulder Elbow. 2016;8(3):171–83. https://doi.org/10.1177/1758573216640210. Epub 2016 Apr 21. PMID: 27583016; PMCID: PMC4950283.
2. Rotini R, Ricciarelli M, Guerra E, Marinelli A, Celli A. Elbow hemiarthroplasty in distal humeral fractures: indication, surgical technique and results. Injury. 2020;54(Suppl 1):S36–45. https://doi.org/10.1016/j.injury.2020.11.020. Epub ahead of print. PMID: 33223259.
3. Phadnis J, Banerjee S, Watts AC, Little N, Hearnden A, Patel VR. Elbow hemiarthroplasty using a "triceps-on" approach for the management of acute distal humeral fractures. J Shoulder Elb Surg. 2015;24(8):1178–86. https://doi.org/10.1016/j.jse.2015.04.010. PMID: 26117619.
4. Celli A, Ricciarelli M, Guerra E, Bonucci P, Ritali A, Cavallo M, Rotini M, Rotini R. Elbow hemiarthroplasty for acute distal humeral fractures and their sequelae: medium- and long-term follow-up of 41 cases. J Shoulder Elb Surg. 2022;31(5):1015–25. https://doi.org/10.1016/j.jse.2021.12.030. Epub 2022 Jan 26. PMID: 35091072.
5. Al-Hamdani A, Rasmussen JV, Sørensen AKB, Ovesen J, Holtz K, Brorson S, Olsen BS. Good outcome after elbow hemiarthroplasty in active patients with an acute intra-articular distal humeral fracture. J Shoulder Elb Surg. 2019;28(5):925–30. https://doi.org/10.1016/j.jse.2018.10.018. Epub 2019 Jan 8. PMID: 30630712.
6. Burkhart KJ, Nijs S, Mattyasovszky SG, Wouters R, Gruszka D, Nowak TE, Rommens PM, Müller LP. Distal humerus hemiarthroplasty of the elbow for comminuted distal humeral fractures in the elderly patient. J Trauma. 2011;71(3):635–42. https://doi.org/10.1097/TA.0b013e318216936e. PMID: 21768901.
7. Chang N, King GJW. Elbow hemiarthroplasty for the treatment of distal humerus fractures. Orthop Clin North Am. 2020;51(2):265–77. https://doi.org/10.1016/j.ocl.2019.11.009. Epub 2020 Feb 3. PMID: 32138864.
8. Nestorson J, Ekholm C, Etzner M, Adolfsson L. Hemiarthroplasty for irreparable distal humeral fractures: medium-term follow-up of 42 patients. Bone Joint J. 2015;97-B(10):1377–84. https://doi.org/10.1302/0301-620X.97B10.35421. PMID: 26430013.
9. Dunn J, Kusnezov N, Pirela-Cruz M. Distal humeral hemiarthroplasty: indications, results, and complications. A systematic review. Hand (NY). 2014;9(4):406–12. https://doi.org/10.1007/s11552-014-9681-3. PMID: 25414601; PMCID: PMC4235903.
10. Jukes CP, Dirckx M, Phadnis J. Current concepts in distal humeral hemiarthroplasty. J Clin Orthop Trauma. 2021;19:224–30. https://doi.org/10.1016/j.jcot.2021.05.025. PMID: 34150495; PMCID: PMC8190472.
11. Guerra E, Zaccaro R, Marinelli A, Cavallo M, Bettelli G, Rotini R. Chapter 5: Surgical approaches for elbow replacements. In: Castoldi F, Giannicola G, Rotini R, editors. Elbow arthroplasty: current techniques and complications. Springer Cham; 2020. p. 57–73.

12. De Vos MJ, Wagener ML, Verdonschot N, Eygendaal D. An extensive posterior approach of the elbow with osteotomy of the medial epicondyle. J Shoulder Elb Surg. 2014;23(3):313–7. https://doi.org/10.1016/j.jse.2013.11.021. PMID: 24524981.
13. Studer A, Athwal GS, MacDermid JC, Faber KJ, King GJ. The lateral para-olecranon approach for total elbow arthroplasty. J Hand Surg Am. 2013;38(11):2219–2226.e3. https://doi.org/10.1016/j.jhsa.2013.07.029. PMID: 24206987.
14. O'Driscoll SW. The triceps-reflecting anconeus pedicle (TRAP) approach for distal humeral fractures and nonunions. Orthop Clin North Am. 2000;31(1):91–101. https://doi.org/10.1016/s0030-5898(05)70130-9. PMID: 10629335.
15. Parsons M, O'Brien RJ, Hughes JS. Elbow hemiarthroplasty for acute and salvage reconstruction of intra-articular distal humerus fractures. Techn Shoulder Elbow Surg. 2005;6(2):87–97.
16. Argintar E, Berry M, Narvy SJ, Kramer J, Omid R, Itamura JM. Hemiarthroplasty for the treatment of distal humerus fractures: short-term clinical results. Orthopedics. 2012;35(12):1042–5.
17. Marinello PG, Peers S, Styron J, Pervaiz K, Evans PJ. Triceps fascial tongue exposure for total elbow arthroplasty: surgical technique and case series. Tech Hand Up Extrem Surg. 2015;19(2):60–3.
18. Na KT, Song SW, Lee YM, Choi JH. Modified triceps fascial tongue approach for primary total elbow arthroplasty. J Shoulder Elb Surg. 2018;27:887–93. https://doi.org/10.1016/j.jse.2018.01.005.
19. Shahane SA, Stanley D. A posterior approach to the elbow joint. J Bone Joint Surg Br. 1999;81(6):1020–2.
20. Weber MB, Cho E, Evans PJ, Styron J, Bafus BT. Triceps tongue versus olecranon osteotomy for intra-articular distal humeral fractures: a matched-cohort study. J Shoulder Elb Surg. 2022;31(6):1215–23.
21. Fei TT, Evans PJ, Bafus BT. Triceps fascial tongue exposure for intra-articular distal humerus fracture: revisiting the Van Gorder approach. JSES Int. 2019;4:39–43. https://doi.org/10.1016/j.jses.2019.10.107.
22. Piggott RP, Hennessy O, Aresti NA. Distal humerus hemiarthroplasty for trauma: a systematic review of the outcomes and complications. J Shoulder Elb Surg. 2022;31(7):1545–52.
23. Wilfred AM, Akhter S, Horner NS, Aljedani A, Khan M, Alolabi B. Outcomes and complications of distal humeral hemiarthroplasty for distal humeral fractures – a systematic review. Shoulder Elbow. 2022;14(1):65–74.

Part III

Hip Arthroplasty

Stefano Zaffagnini

8 Patient Position and General Setting in Total Hip Arthroplasty

F. Raggi, T. Cerasoli, D. Alesi, Giulio Maria Marcheggiani Muccioli, M. Zaffagnini, E. Tassinari, and Stefano Zaffagnini

8.1 Introduction

Total hip arthroplasty (THA) is one of the most successful and cost-effective orthopedics surgeries. It provides reliable and enduring outcomes for patients suffering from end-stage degenerative hip osteoarthritis, congenital hip disorders, avascular necrosis of femoral head, inflammatory diseases, and trauma sequelae [1, 2]. Studies conducted in the United States have projected an almost 200% increase in the demand for total hip arthroplasty by 2030 based on current rates. Various surgical approaches exist for THA, the most frequently performed being the direct lateral, posterior, and direct anterior approaches [3]. While each approach retains its distinct characteristics, a common thread among them all is the critical emphasis on the precise positioning of patients. The efficacy of the procedure hinges on meticulous patient positioning, optimal pelvis' alignment, and stability throughout the surgical process. This chapter is dedicated to understanding the importance of patient positioning and the overall setup in the context of THA in the three most frequently performed approaches.

F. Raggi (✉) · T. Cerasoli · D. Alesi · G. M. Marcheggiani Muccioli · M. Zaffagnini · E. Tassinari · S. Zaffagnini
IRCCS Istituto Ortopedico Rizzoli, University of Bologna, Bologna, Italy
e-mail: federico.raggi@ior.it

G. M. Marcheggiani Muccioli et al. (eds.), *Easy Planning in Elective Primary Orthopedic Procedures*, https://doi.org/10.1007/978-3-031-77006-7_8

8.2 Anesthesia

Various anesthetic and analgesic approaches have been explored for THA, but the optimal technique remains a topic of debate. While general anesthesia has traditionally been considered the "gold standard" for most hip procedures due to its rapid and comprehensive effects, postoperative pain management, length of stay, and associated healthcare costs suggest the need for alternative approaches [4, 5]. Regional anesthesia stands out as a favorable option, providing superior intraoperative and postoperative pain control, reducing opioid use, shortening recovery time, and decreasing the length of hospital stay. It also correlates with lower incidence of complications such as deep vein thrombosis, hypoxemia, pulmonary issues, intraoperative blood loss, and postoperative confusion [4, 6–9, 10].

Among regional techniques, spinal anesthesia (or subarachnoid anesthesia) is the most used. It is a simple and swift technique, showing better outcomes than general anesthesia. However, it poses risks of severe hypotension and has a limited duration of action. To overcome these limitations, its variants such as unilateral spinal anesthesia or a combination of spinal with epidural anesthesia were introduced, obtaining denser and longer-lasting blocks with reduced hypotension, prolonged analgesia, faster onset, and lower failure rates [4, 5]. Combined sciatic nerve/lumbar plexus block with general sedation has proven effective, less invasive, and more selective for THA patients, especially in the elderly or those with comorbidities, without impacting postoperative analgesic consumption, mortality rates, or hospital stays [7]. Recently, other regional techniques have gained prominence. Suprainguinal fascia iliaca block rivals lumbar plexus block in pain control and opioid consumption but may decrease motor strength, delaying postoperative mobilization. The pericapsular nerve group (PENG) block selectively targets articular branches, sparing motor components allowing early postoperative mobilization, at the cost of less patient relaxation with potential difficulties in intraoperative maneuvers [11].

Considering multiple perioperative outcomes, there is a consensus that spinal anesthesia is the preferred technique (when no contraindications exist), reducing the risk of most complications [9, 10].

8.3 Patient Positioning

Proper patient positioning for THA is essential to optimize implant positioning, monitor limb length discrepancies and facilitate surgical intervention. Two different patient positions (lateral and supine decubitus) have been proposed, depending on the surgical approach (direct anterior, direct lateral, and posterolateral) and the surgeon's preference. While the direct anterior and direct lateral approaches can be performed in both positions, the posterolateral approach is only feasible in lateral decubitus [12, 13].

It is crucial to understand that the patient's positioning in THA significantly influences the placement of prosthetic components, especially after draping when the pelvis is no longer directly visible to the surgeon. Therefore, the patient should be positioned correctly, and the position should be stabilized on the operating table, as maneuvers such as dislocating the native hip and using retractors can cause intraoperative pelvic movement, altering pelvic orientation with potential disastrous effects on the placement of prosthetic components [13, 14]. After preparing the surgical field and covering pelvic landmarks (anterior superior iliac spines), the surgeon's only way to precisely orient themselves in case of patient mispositioning is through fluoroscopy. Therefore, it is preferable to use radiolucent beds to allow for intraoperative checks if needed. Once anesthesia is completed, the patients' genitals are covered with sterile gauze and sterile drapes before starting the patient positioning on the operating table.

In lateral decubitus, the patient is placed with the hip to be operated on the top. A pad should be positioned under the knee of the limb not undergoing surgery to prevent peroneal nerve neuropraxia, and the limb should be secured to the bed with a gentle bandage, flexed at 30–45°. During patient positioning, another pad should be placed between the knees to prevent pressure ulcers, and both legs are kept on the bed with a security belt to facilitate the other maneuvers. To maintain the patient's position and support the pelvis, pads are placed on the front over the superior iliac spines and one on the back over the sacrum. One additional pad is positioned on the back to support the patient (Fig. 8.1).

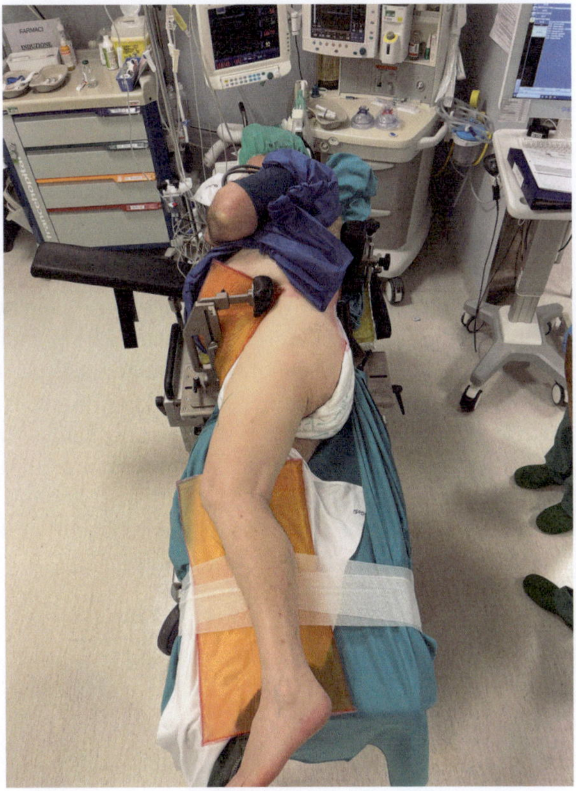

Fig. 8.1 Preoperative patient positioning in lateral decubitus

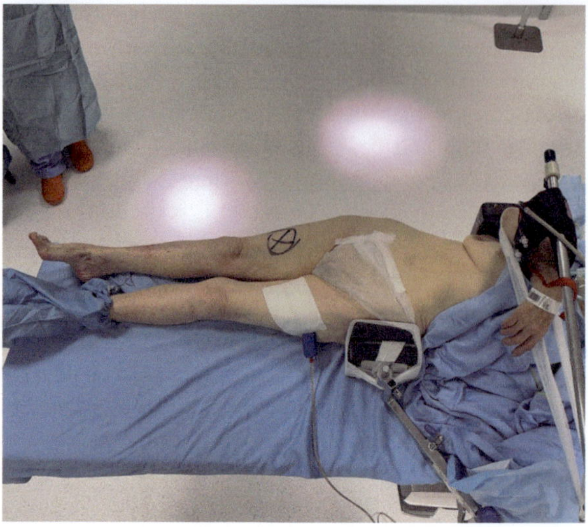

Fig. 8.2 Preoperative patient positioning in supine decubitus

The patient's pelvis should be perpendicular to the bed. To ensure the patient's stability and prevent the pads from hindering intraoperative maneuvers, it is crucial to test the planned maneuvers before draping. Specifically, the pads must allow for a flexion of the operated hip of at least 100°. The patient's arm in contact with the bed is left free, while the arm above can be gently placed on the patient's torso or positioned with the shoulder at a 90° flexion over a support or bolster with appropriate padding [12, 13, 15]. This position is recommended for obese patients. In the lateral position, the fatty tissue falls away from the surgical field, this allows for proper visualization and hemostasis [15].

In the supine decubitus, the patient is positioned flat on the table with the pelvis held horizontally and not inclined. The hip intended for surgery is placed at the lateral edge of the bed, allowing the buttock muscles and gluteal fat to fall posteriorly away from the operative plane. This positioning enhances the view of the acetabular cavity, facilitates femoral exposure during adduction and external rotation, and optimizes the placement of retractors. A pad is positioned on the opposite hip to stabilize the pelvis, and another pad is placed on the side to be operated at the thoracic level to provide additional stabilization. Limbs should be securely fastened to the bed using a seatbelt during patient positioning. The arm on the nonoperative side can be on a support outside the operating bed. The arm on the operative side can be positioned on the patient's chest, or over a support or bolster with appropriate padding with the shoulder at a 90° flexion (Fig. 8.2) [12, 13, 15].

8.4 Surgical Preparation and Draping

To minimize the risk of surgical site infection, antibiotic prophylaxis (primarily using second-generation cephalosporins) should be administered 30–60 min before making the skin incision [16]. Once the patient is positioned on the operating table, the surgical area's skin is cleaned with a 4.0% chlorhexidine gluconate solution. Alternatively, povidone-iodine (Betadine) can be used, but it has demonstrated lower efficacy in reducing surgical site infections in total hip arthroplasty (THA) when applied to the skin. However, when it is used for the lavage of wounds before closure plays an essential role in minimizing infection risk in THA. This is because it has the ability to inhibit biofilm production by organisms such as *Staphylococcus epidermidis* and *Staphylococcus aureus*, which are among the most frequently implicated pathogens [17, 16].

In the lateral decubitus, the leg to be operated is released from the securing belt that held it on the bed, and the pad between the legs is removed. The nonoperative leg is maintained in the previously fixed position. An unscrubbed assistant lifts the leg to be operated from the foot, and two scrubbed operators completely disinfect it with chlorhexidine. The disinfection starts from the hip, moving upward to the abdomen at the level of the navel, and downward to the ankle. The operators step away from the surgical field while the leg is kept elevated, and the scrub nurse positions a large sterile drape to prevent the surgeons from touching the operating table during the foot disinfection. One surgeon holds the disinfected leg using sterile gauze from the ankle, and the foot is disinfected. The third operator puts on the impermeable stockinette on the foot and unrolls it up to above the knee. The stockinette is then covered and secured with a disposable elastic wrap (such as an Esmark). Since the drape will not adhere to the skin when it is wet, the hip area should be dried with a sterile towel before draping if it is still wet. Three drapes are placed anteriorly, posteriorly, and proximally to the surgical site, and an impermeable reinforced U-shaped drape is positioned inferiorly to the leg to be operated, covering the other drapes. The leg is then led onto the surgical field. The head drape is positioned proximally to the incision site over the U-shaped drape. To minimize the risk of surgeons touching any non-sterile components during the dislocation and reduction maneuvers, one large sterile drape is placed above the U-shaped drape under the patient's leg, and one is positioned medially and one laterally from the incision site. At last, an adhesive transparent drape is placed to cover completely the skin of the surgical site (Fig. 8.3).

In the supine decubitus, there are two different ways to draping depending on the surgical technique. When a direct lateral approach is chosen, only the leg to be operated is included in the surgical field. An unscrubbed assistant maintains the leg to be operated flexed and adducted to allow for the disinfection of the hip, buttock, and abdomen up to the navel. While keeping the leg flexed and adducted, the scrub nurse positions a sterile approach drape under the buttock and the side. At this point, the unscrubbed assistant lifts the leg from the ankle, and two operators continue to paint it with chlorhexidine down to the ankle. One operator lifts the leg from the ankle using sterile gauzes, allowing the scrub nurse to position a large sterile drape over

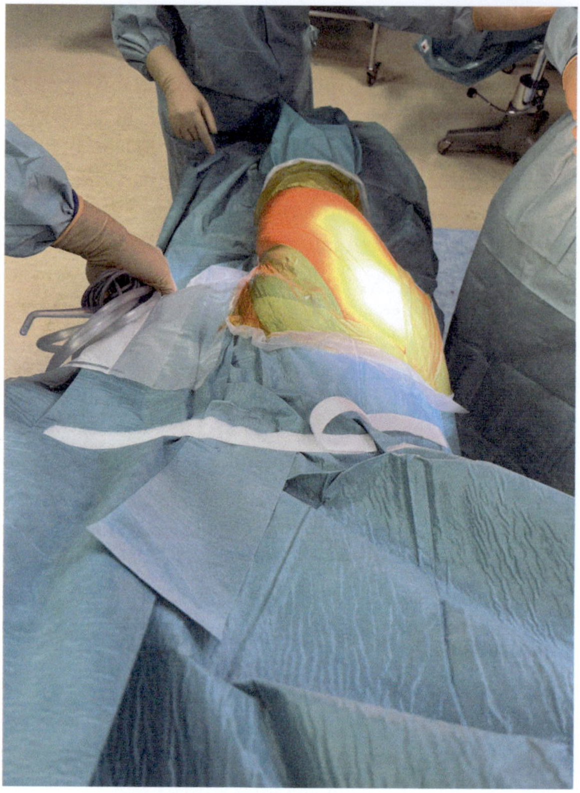

Fig. 8.3 Ultimate surgical draping for patient in lateral decubitus

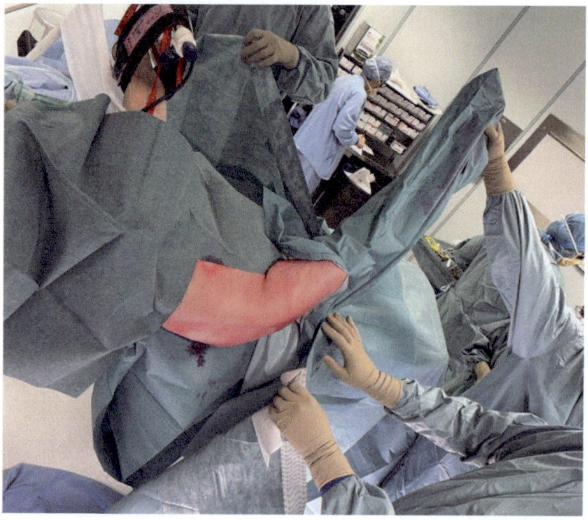

Fig. 8.4 Correct positioning of the stockinette under the U-shaped sterile drape

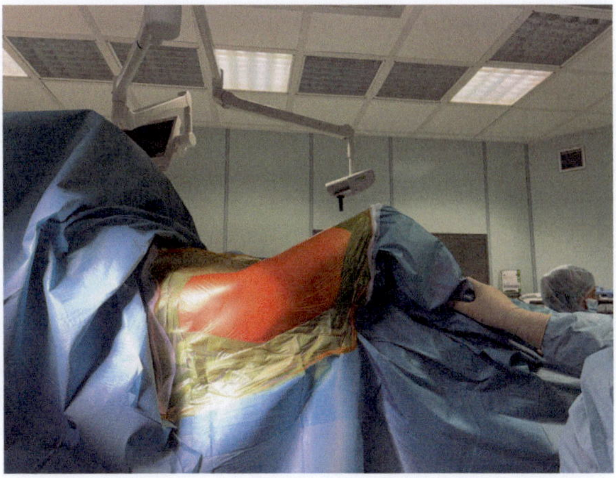

Fig. 8.5 Ultimate surgical draping for patient in lateral decubitus when direct lateral surgical approach is chosen

the nonoperative leg, excluding it from the surgical field. The surgeons complete the disinfection of the foot and position the stockinette, holding the operative leg from the ankle. Two sterile drapes are placed, one medial and one proximal to the surgical site. The stockinette is unrolled up to above the knee and cut laterally so that the lower edge can rest on the underlying drapes (Fig. 8.4).

A U-shaped sterile drape is positioned passing under the leg to be operated and over the distal edges of the stockinette and other pads. Finally, the head drape and two drapes, one medial and one lateral, are placed to minimize the risk of the operators touching anything non-sterile. While keeping the leg flexed at approximately 30° and adducted, an adhesive transparent drape is positioned on the skin and the proximal end of the stockinette completing the surgical field (Fig. 8.5).

When a direct anterior approach is chosen, both legs should be included in the surgical field to allow for maintaining the abducted and externally rotated position of the femur achieved by placing the operative leg under the other, as well as to facilitate easy monitoring of limb length. Two unscrubbed assistants lift the legs by holding them at the feet. The operators disinfect the limbs from the abdomen to the level of the navel down to the ankles, then they lift the legs from the ankles using sterile gauzes. The scrub nurse places a sterile drape to cover the operating table. The surgeons complete the disinfection of the feet. Two stockinettes are positioned, and the legs are kept elevated and abducted from the ankles. A proximal drape is placed at the level of the abdomen just distal to the navel. Subsequently, the scrub nurse positions a W-shaped drape with perineal coverage. At this point, the stockinettes are unrolled up to above the knee and secured with an elastic wrap (such as an Esmark). Both limbs are thus included in the surgical field. The head drape and two lateral drapes are positioned to isolated the hip that will not be operated, and minimize the risk of the operators touching anything non-sterile. An adhesive transparent drape is positioned on the skin and the proximal end of the stockinette completing the surgical field.

The direct anterior approach can also be performed using a traction table to facilitate exposure of the femoral head. The patient is placed supine with the limb to be operated tethered to traction using a leg holder. The other leg lies supine on the surgical table, and a perineal post is positioned between the legs. The leg to be operated is slightly adducted, with the hip slightly flexed. An unscrubbed assistant will handle leg traction throughout the procedure, ensuring to stay under the sterile drapes. The operators disinfect the limbs from the abdomen down to the level of the navel, extending to the beginning of the leg holder. The scrub nurse places a sterile drape to cover from the knee downward. A proximal drape is positioned at the level of the abdomen just distal to the navel. The operators place three pads to demarcate the surgical area: one proximal to the navel, one medial to cover the perineal post, and one lateral. Subsequently, they position a U-shaped drape above the three pads, leaving the knee in the operating field. Afterward, the head drape is positioned. An adhesive transparent drape is placed on the skin and the proximal end of the U-shaped drape, completing the surgical field.

8.5 Operating Room Layout

The operating room should accommodate four surgeons at the operating table, along with the scrub nurse, anesthesiologist, and operating room nurse. Additionally, it must allow for the entry and positioning of the fluoroscopy device if intraoperative checks are necessary. There are two doors: the main entrance remains closed during surgery to minimize staff traffic, while the second door opens to the scrubbing area [17]. Anesthesia equipment and the anesthesiologist are located at the head of the patient. Power sources, cautery generators, and suction tubing are also located at the head of the patient. Within the operating room, two Mayo stands are positioned on the operating side of the patient, right behind the first and second operators and the scrub nurse. One Mayo stand accommodates mobile shelving units containing common sets of implants, while the other holds mobile shelving units with specific prosthetic equipment. The operating table is directly beneath the operating lights and the laminar flow [17]. The primary light is positioned above the right shoulder of the dominant surgeon, while the secondary light is above the right shoulder of the second operator. A computer may be available in the operating room for reviewing preoperative digital imaging.

8.6 Surgical Team Layout

The anesthesiologist is located at the head of the operating table. The first operator is positioned in front of the surgical site when the patient is supine (Figs. 8.6, 8.7) and behind the patient when he is in a lateral decubitus position (Fig. 8.8). The second operator is beside the first operator on the side of the patient's head. When an

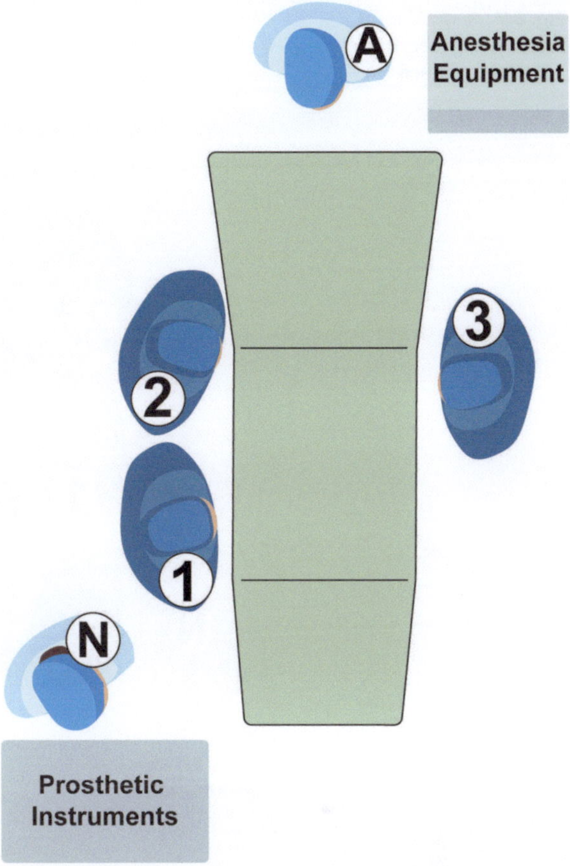

Fig. 8.6 Surgical team layout when direct anterior approach is chosen

anterior approach or a posterior approach is chosen, the third operator is located in front of the first surgeon. When a lateral approach is chosen, the third operator is positioned at the patient's leg, and a fourth operator is in front of the first surgeon, holding the retractors in place (Fig. 8.7). The scrub nurse stands on the operative side of the patient right behind the first surgeon.

Take Home Messages

1. Proper patient positioning in THA is crucial to optimize implant placement, monitor limb length, and facilitate surgical intervention, particularly after draping when the pelvis is no longer directly visible to the surgeon.
2. Two distinct patient positions (lateral or supine decubitus) are proposed based on surgical and surgeon preference.
3. In the supine position, ensure the patient's pelvis is held horizontally and not inclined. The hip designated for surgery should be positioned at the lateral edge

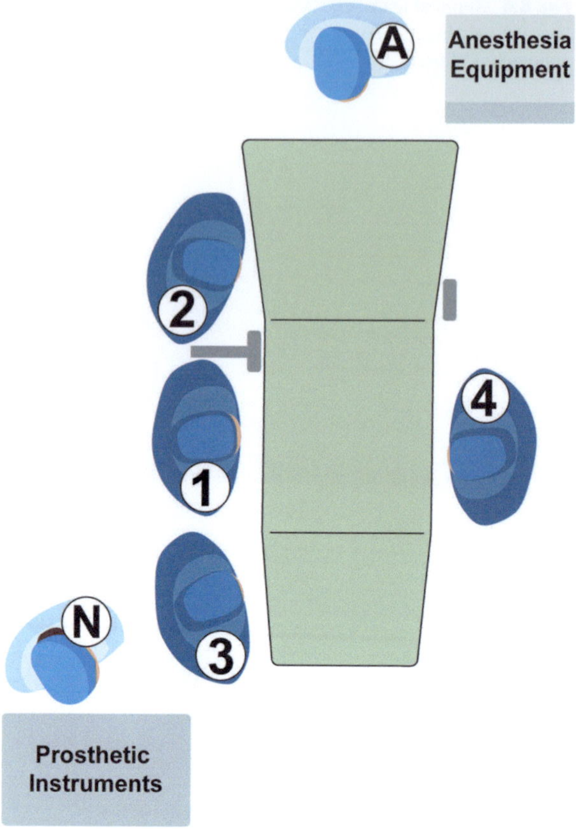

Fig. 8.7 Surgical team layout when direct lateral approach is chosen

of the bed, allowing the buttock muscles and gluteal fat to fall posteriorly away from the operative plane.

4. During lateral decubitus, secure the patient's pelvis perpendicular to the bed using two pads that do not impede intraoperative maneuvers.
5. To minimize the risk of postoperative infection, it is crucial to perform appropriate skin disinfection and draping based on the surgical technique.
6. Avoid inadequate padding of bony prominences may lead to neuropraxia.

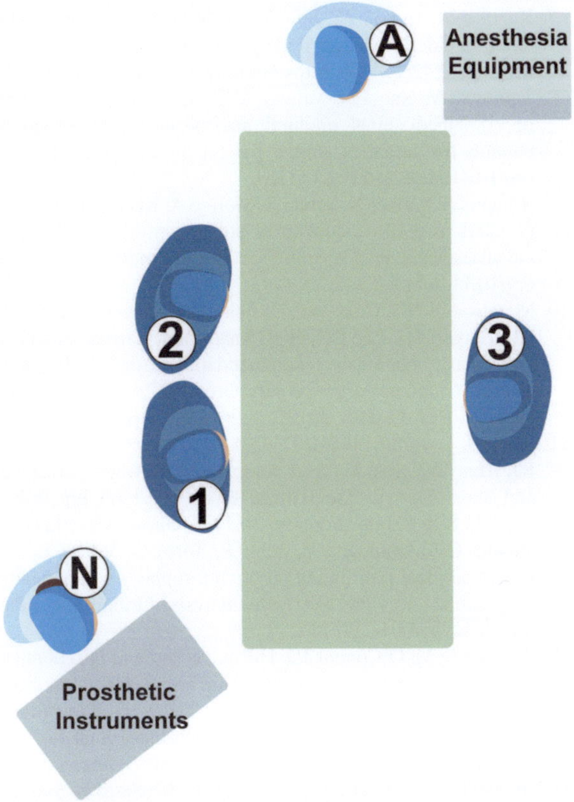

Fig. 8.8 Surgical team layout when posterolateral approach is chosen

References

1. Varacallo M, Luo TD, Johanson NA. Total hip arthroplasty techniques. Treasure Island, FL: StatPearls Publishing; 2023.
2. Kumar P, Sen RK, Aggarwal S, Jindal K. Common hip conditions requiring primary total hip arthroplasty and comparison of their post-operative functional outcomes. J Clin Orthop Trauma. 2020;11:S192–5. https://doi.org/10.1016/j.jcot.2019.02.009.
3. Talia AJ, Coetzee C, Tirosh O, Tran P. Comparison of outcome measures and complication rates following three different approaches for primary total hip arthroplasty: a pragmatic randomised controlled trial. Trials. 2018;19:13. https://doi.org/10.1186/s13063-017-2368-7.
4. Liang C, Wei J, Cai X, Lin W, Fan Y, Yang F. Efficacy and safety of 3 different anesthesia techniques used in total hip arthroplasty. Med Sci Monit Int Med J Exp Clin Res. 2017;23:3752–9. https://doi.org/10.12659/msm.902768.
5. Magar JS, Bawdane KD, Patil R. Comparison of efficacy and safety of unilateral spinal anaesthesia with sequential combined spinal epidural anaesthesia for lower limb orthopaedic surgery. J Clin Diagn Res. 2017;11:UC17–UC20. https://doi.org/10.7860/JCDR/2017/26235.10215.
6. Pu X, Sun J-M. General anesthesia vs spinal anesthesia for patients undergoing Total-hip arthroplasty: a meta-analysis. Medicine (Baltimore). 2019;98:e14925. https://doi.org/10.1097/MD.0000000000014925.

7. Kaçmaz M, Turhan ZY. Spinal anesthesia versus combined sciatic nerve/lumbar plexus nerve block in elderly patients undergoing total hip arthroplasty: a retrospective study. Ann Saudi Med. 2022;42:174–80. https://doi.org/10.5144/0256-4947.2022.174.
8. Tummala V, Rao LN, Vallury MK, Sanapala A. A comparative study-efficacy and safety of combined spinal epidural anesthesia versus spinal anesthesia in high-risk geriatric patients for surgeries around the hip joint. Anesth Essays Res. 2015;9:185–8. https://doi.org/10.4103/0259-1162.153764.
9. Rodgers A, Walker N, Schug S, McKee A, Kehlet H, van Zundert A, Sage D, Futter M, Saville G, Clark T, et al. Reduction of postoperative mortality and morbidity with epidural or spinal anaesthesia: results from overview of randomised trials. BMJ. 2000;321:1493. https://doi.org/10.1136/bmj.321.7275.1493.
10. Memtsoudis SG, Cozowicz C, Bekeris J, Bekere D, Liu J, Soffin EM, Mariano ER, Johnson RL, Hargett MJ, Lee BH, et al. Anaesthetic care of patients undergoing primary hip and knee arthroplasty: consensus recommendations from the International Consensus on Anaesthesia-Related Outcomes after Surgery Group (ICAROS) based on a systematic review and meta-analysis. Br J Anaesth. 2019;123:269–87. https://doi.org/10.1016/j.bja.2019.05.042.
11. Aliste J, Layera S, Bravo D, Jara Á, Muñoz G, Barrientos C, Wulf R, Brañez J, Finlayson RJ, Tran DQ. Randomized comparison between pericapsular Nerve Group (PENG) block and suprainguinal fascia iliaca block for total hip arthroplasty. Reg Anesth Pain Med. 2021;46:874–8. https://doi.org/10.1136/rapm-2021-102997.
12. Papalia GF, Zampogna B, Albo E, Torre G, Villari E, Papalia R, Denaro V. The role of patient surgical positioning on hip arthroplasty component placement and clinical outcomes: a systematic re-view and meta-analysis. Orthop Rev (Pavia). 2023;15:74116. https://doi.org/10.52965/001c.74116.
13. Rutherford M, O'Connor JD, Hill JC, Beverland DE, Lennon AB, Dunne NJ. Patient positioning and cup orientation during total hip arthroplasty: assessment of current UK practice. Hip Int J Clin Exp Res Hip Pathol Ther. 2019;29:89–95. https://doi.org/10.1177/1120700018760818.
14. Noordin S, Lakdawala R, Masri BA. Primary total hip arthroplasty: staying out of trouble intraoperatively. Ann Med Surg. 2018;29:30–3. https://doi.org/10.1016/j.amsu.2018.03.043.
15. Hoppenfeld, S.; DeBoer, P.; Buckley, R. (Richard E. Surgical exposures in orthopaedics : the anatomic approach; 5th.; Wolters Kluwer: Philadelphia, 2016.; ISBN 1-4963-7360-X.
16. Tarabichi S, Parvizi J. Prevention of surgical site infection: a ten-step approach. Arthroplast (London, England). 2023;5:21. https://doi.org/10.1186/s42836-023-00174-7.
17. Dobson PF, Reed MR. Prevention of infection in primary THA and TKA. EFORT Open Rev. 2020;5:604–13. https://doi.org/10.1302/2058-5241.5.200004.

Preoperative Planning for Primary Total Hip Arthroplasty

9

F. Raggi, D. Alesi, M. Zaffagnini, M. Casali, Giulio Maria Marcheggiani Muccioli, M. Romagnoli, and Stefano Zaffagnini

9.1 Introduction

Preoperative planning is a fundamental aspect of reestablishing native biomechanics of the hip in total hip arthroplasty (THA). In the literature, many authors discuss the importance of preoperative X-ray review and measurement to establish the correct positioning of the implant components [1–3]. Hip replacement surgery aims to restore the center of rotation of the coxofemoral articulation and femoral offset, focusing on equalizing limb length. Another important point is the opportunity for surgeons to evaluate the hip anatomy and estimate the implant sizes with a high level of precision [4–7]. When the preoperative planning coincides with intraoperative limb-length measurement, the incidence of dysmetria of lower limbs significantly decreases [8, 9], although mild dysmetria does not affect the patient's outcome [10, 11].

The patient's sex, age, hip anatomy, hip disease, medical history, level of activity, and expectations from the surgery need to be considered when choosing the type and design of the prosthesis.

With the advent of technology, surgeons have reduced the use of printed radiograph films, and templating is now done with computer software. However, traditional templating with X-rays continues to be a good possible option. This chapter will describe an accurate and reproducible technique of preoperative radiograph templating for THA.

F. Raggi (✉) · D. Alesi · M. Zaffagnini · M. Casali · G. M. Marcheggiani Muccioli · M. Romagnoli · S. Zaffagnini
IRCCS Istituto Ortopedico Rizzoli, University of Bologna, Bologna, Italy
e-mail: federico.raggi@ior.it

G. M. Marcheggiani Muccioli et al. (eds.), *Easy Planning in Elective Primary Orthopedic Procedures*, https://doi.org/10.1007/978-3-031-77006-7_9

9.2 Radiographic Evaluation

Preoperative templating should be done using a standard anteroposterior (AP) radiograph of the pelvis. The correct positioning of the patients and the tube-to-film distance are crucial. The AP pelvis film is traditionally taken supine to prevent any possible pelvic obliquity caused by leg length discrepancy. The weight-bearing position has also been used in recent years, according to the advances in human spinopelvic kinematics [12]. It should be centered on the symphysis pubis with a standard magnification that could be reproduced every time and a magnification marker [13]. The legs of the patient have to be positioned internally rotated of 15°. A perfect radiograph has to show the symmetry of the lesser trochanters and the obturator foramen [14] (Fig. 9.1).

9.3 Templating Technique

Leg length discrepancy is evaluated by drawing the interdrope line or trans-ischial reference line, noting where they intersect the lesser trochanters (Fig. 9.2) [15–17].

A detailed physical examination is also necessary to confirm the cause of dysmetria. It may be caused by a hip disease or pelvic obliquity, caused by scoliosis, or rheumatic disease of the spine. If there is a pelvic obliquity, it is not possible to resolve leg length discrepancy with a THA.

However, joint contractures can also interfere with clinical leg length assessment; the surgeon has to rule out this possibility with a clinical test like the Thomas test for iliopsoas contracture. Moreover, in pelvis X-rays, it is possible to observe signs of acetabular retroversion such as crossover signs, posterior wall signs, and prominence of the ischial spine [18].

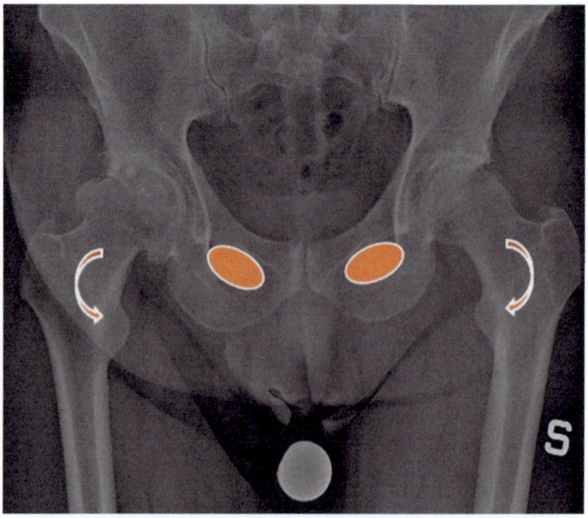

Fig. 9.1 Example of a good pelvic radiograph for planning. The symmetry of foramen obturatorum, same femur intrarotation, magnification marker

Fig. 9.2 Interdrope line or trans-ischial reference line and the distance from the apex of the lesser trochanter

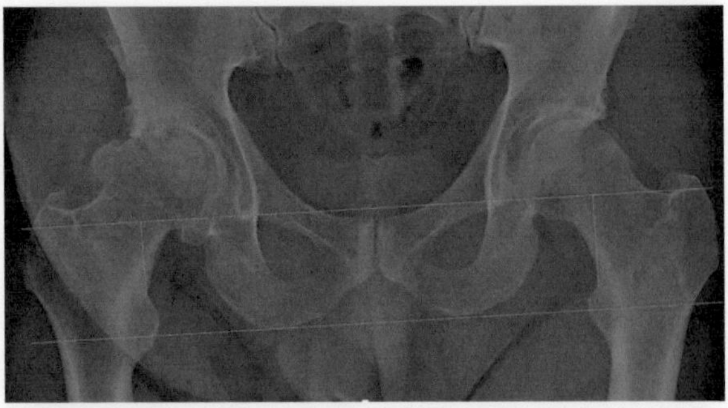

Fig. 9.3 Identification of the ideal CoR of the hip

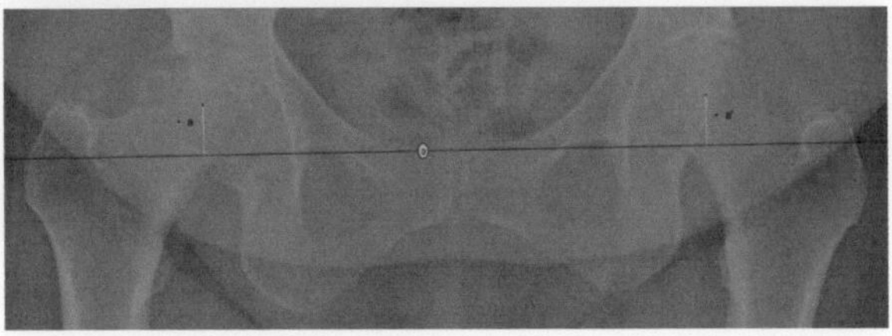

The goal of the templating of the acetabulum is to restore the hip center of rotation (CoR) to premorbidity or previous anatomic location. To achieve this goal, the CoR of the healthy hip is marked, which is speculated on the pathological side using the longitudinal axis as the axis of symmetry (Fig. 9.3).

The ideal CoR of the acetabular cup should coincide with the newly traced one. However, if a compromise is necessary, the CoR can be moved along the green line while maintaining the 45° angle or within the dial bounded by the two green lines, which define the safety zone (Fig. 9.4).

In the past, templating was achieved by using traditional systems (manual planning with slides) (Fig. 9.5).

Nowadays, dedicated software is available worldwide and allows bidimensional (2D) planning on standard X-rays (this kind of templating is described in the present paragraph). In complex cases, such as obese patients, hip dysplasia, protusio acetabuli, and in revision THA, restoring the correct center of rotation is difficult with both systems, whereas modern software utilizing 3D templating is useful to obtain better accuracy [19, 20]. A 2D templating can not give information to the surgeon about the anteversion of the acetabulum and the femur, contrary to tridimensional (3D) templating software such as HIP-OP and ZEDHIP [21, 22]. Bony landmarks are teardrop, superolateral acetabular margin, and Kohler line. The acetabulum should be covered completely by bone, centered under the column of the ilium, usually medialized to the lateral wall of the teardrop, matching the arc of the superolateral acetabular margin (Fig. 9.6).

The acetabular inclination should be placed in the safe zone of Lewinnek (abduction 40° ± 10°; anteversion 15° ± 10°) [23]. A lower inclination of the cup decreases

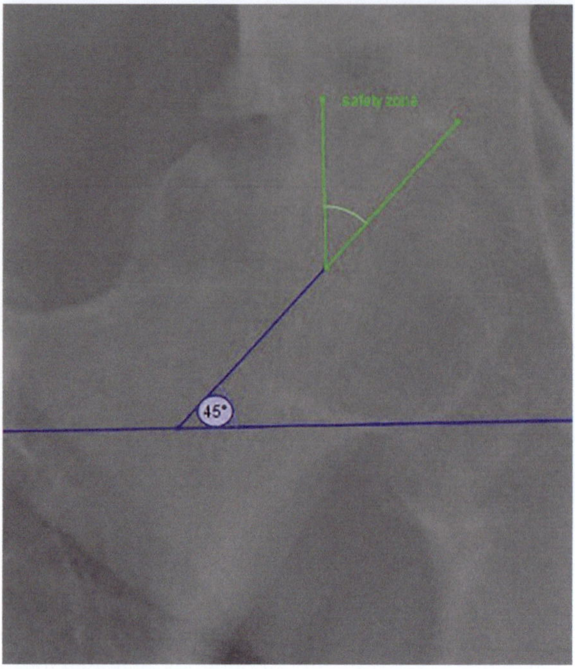

Fig. 9.4 Safety zone

abduction of the hip; however, a higher abduction increases the risk of dislocation and wear of the polyethylene liner of the prosthesis [24].

The femoral component is templated to restore the patient's leg length and lateral and vertical offset.

First of all, check the morphology and bone quality of the proximal femur in the X-rays of the pelvis. Use the classification of Dorr or the Canal Flare Index to predict and reduce the risk of intraoperative fracture of the femoral neck (Tables 9.1 and 9.2) [25–28].

For example, in type C of Dorr classification, think about the possibility of a cemented stem. Moreover, consider the design of the stem according to the Canal Flare Index; in a Champagne-Flute, consider a metaphyseal stem, while in a stovepipe, a diaphyseal stem (Fig. 9.7).

The stem should be centered for the bone envelope, selecting the most appropriate size (Fig. 9.8). It may be useful to calculate the cut distance (CD) preoperatively. Before performing the femoral neck resection (FNR), measure with a caliber the CD, which must match the preoperative measure. Therefore, draw a landmark on the bone and proceed with the FNR. Moreover, the preoperative sinking of the stem (B) must be measured intraoperatively with the definitive stem caliber. Those measures must match to restore exactly the limb lengths as templating in the preoperative planning (Fig. 9.2). Moreover, in a lower femoral neck-shaft angle (coxa vara), consider an increased lateral offset to restore the native biomechanics of the hip

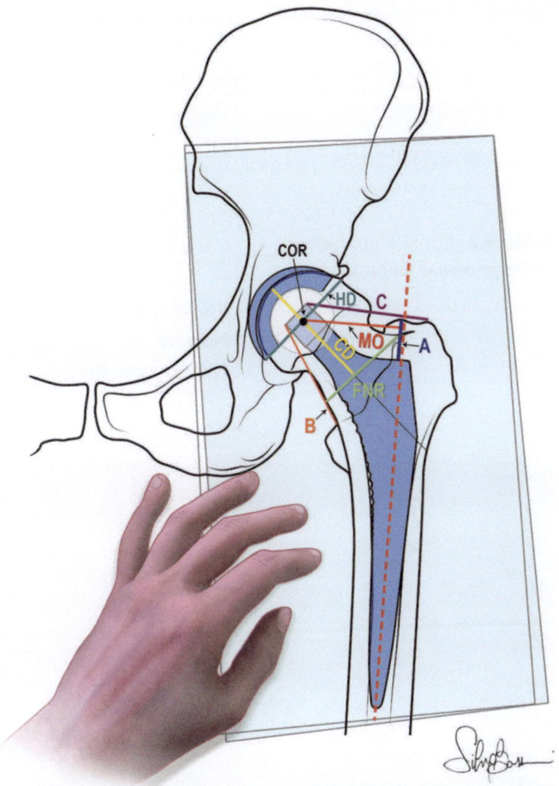

Fig. 9.5 Manual planning: overlaying of the prosthesis slides to the native X-ray. One slide represents the acetabular and liner components, and the other the stem component. (A) sinking of the stem from the greater trochanter; (B) sinking from the tip of the stem to the lesser trochanter; (C) distance from the tip of the stem to the greater trochanter; *CD* cut distance; *COR* center of rotation; *FNR* femoral neck resection; *HD* head diameter; *MO* medial offset. Copyright of Silvia Bassini, 2024. All rights reserved

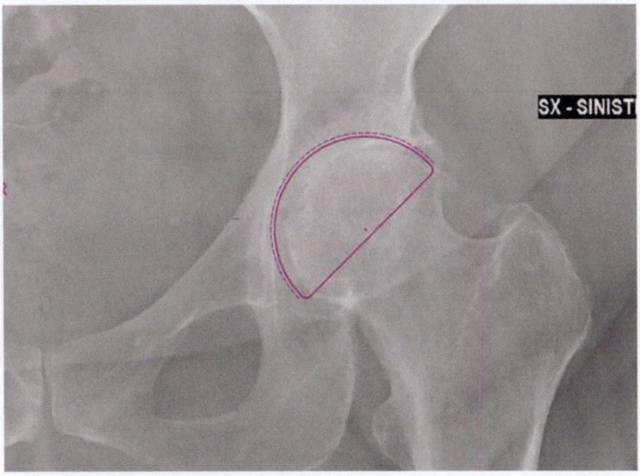

Fig. 9.6 The cup acetabular component is templated in the anatomic position

Table 9.1 Dorr classification of the proximal femur [25]

Dorr classification	
	Ratio
Type A	<0.5
Type B	0.5–0.75
Type C	>0.75

Table 9.2 Canal Flare Index of the proximal femur [26]

Canal Flare Index	
	Ratio
Stovepipe	<3.0
Normal	3.0–4.7
Champagne-flute	>4.7

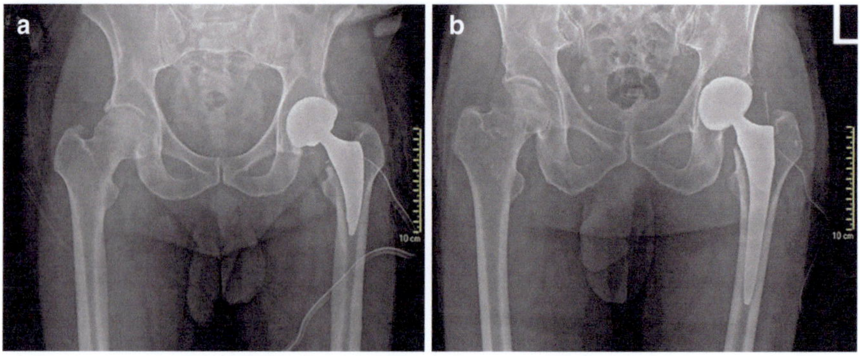

Fig. 9.7 (**a**) Metaphyseal stem in a Champagne-Flute canal shape. (**b**) Diaphyseal stem in a stovepipe canal shape

Fig. 9.8 The stem femur component is templated in the anatomic position, centered for the bone envelope, and selected to the most appropriate size

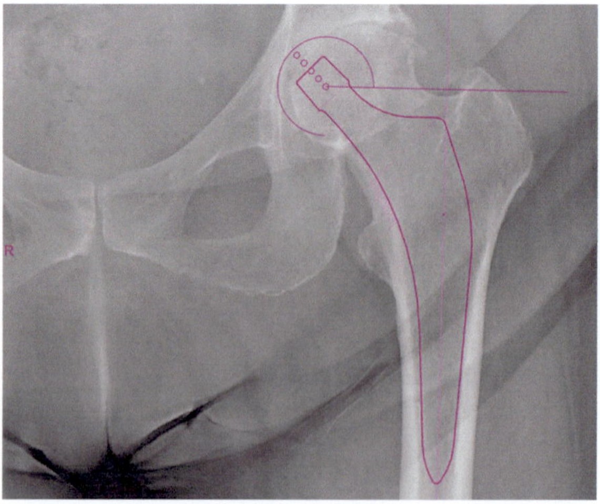

patient. Remember that decreasing the femoral offset may lead to a higher polyethylene wear rate [29–32].

The depth of insertion is important to restore leg length. Choose a bigger size to increase leg length, conversely, a smaller to decrease leg length. Furthermore, the size of femoral heads should be maximus whenever possible because of an increased risk of impingement and instability [33].

The level of femoral neck resection depends on the type of stems used [34]. Lesser trochanters are intraoperative landmarks that are easily identifiable. Measure the distance from the superior margin of the lesser trochanter to the neck resection template. It should be matched during surgery when the trial stem is implanted.

Take Home Message

1. The systematic use of preoperative templating is fundamental for the THA implantation.
2. Preoperative planning must be reproducible; it is a guide before and during surgery, and it shortens operative time.
3. Intraoperative checks reduce deviation from preoperative planning and also help in recognizing an intraoperative mistake when a large discrepancy exists between a trial component and the template [4].

References

1. Colombi A, Schena D, Castelli CC. Total hip arthroplasty planning. EFORT Open Rev. 2019;4:626–32.
2. Bishi H, et al. Comparison of the accuracy of 2D and 3D templating methods for planning primary total hip replacement: a systematic review and meta-analysis. EFORT Open Rev. 2022;7:70–83.
3. Della Valle AG, Padgett DE, Salvati EA. Preoperative planning for primary total hip arthroplasty. J Am Acad Orthop Surg. 2005;13:455–62.
4. Shaarani SR, McHugh G, Collins DA. Accuracy of digital preoperative templating in 100 consecutive uncemented total hip arthroplasties: a single surgeon series. J Arthroplast. 2013;28:331–7.
5. Eggli S, Pisan M, Müller ME. The value of preoperative planning for total hip arthroplasty. J Bone Joint Surg Br. 1998;80:382–90.
6. Wedemeyer C, et al. Digital templating in total hip arthroplasty with the Mayo stem. Arch Orthop Trauma Surg. 2008;128:1023–9.
7. Davila JA, Kransdorf MJ, Duffy GP. Surgical planning of total hip arthroplasty: accuracy of computer-assisted EndoMap software in predicting component size. Skeletal Radiol. 2006;35:390–3.
8. Woolson ST. Leg length equalization during total hip replacement. Orthopedics. 1990;13:17–21.
9. Abraham WD, Dimon JH. Leg length discrepancy in total hip arthroplasty. Orthop Clin North Am. 1992;23:201–9.
10. Mahmood SS, Mukka SS, Crnalic S, Sayed-Noor AS. The influence of leg length discrepancy after Total hip arthroplasty on function and quality of life: a prospective cohort study. J Arthroplast. 2015;30:1638–42.

11. Ng VY, Kean JR, Glassman AH. Limb-length discrepancy after hip arthroplasty. J Bone Joint Surg Am. 2013;95:1426–36.
12. DelSole EM, Mercuri JJ. Utility of upright weight-bearing imaging in total hip arthroplasty. Semin Musculoskelet Radiol. 2019;23:603–8.
13. Conn KS, Clarke MT, Hallett JP. A simple guide to determine the magnification of radiographs and to improve the accuracy of preoperative templating. J Bone Joint Surg Br. 2002;84:269–72.
14. Kate BR. Anteversion versus torsion of the femoral neck. Acta Anat (Basel). 1976;94:457–63.
15. Tipton SC, Sutherland JK, Schwarzkopf R. The assessment of limb length discrepancy before total hip arthroplasty. J Arthroplast. 2016;31:888–92.
16. McWilliams AB, et al. Assessing reproducibility for radiographic measurement of leg length inequality after total hip replacement. Hip Int. 2012;22:539–44.
17. Meermans G, Malik A, Witt J, Haddad F. Preoperative radiographic assessment of limb-length discrepancy in total hip arthroplasty. Clin Orthop Relat Res. 2011;469:1677–82.
18. Kappe T, et al. Reliability of radiographic signs for acetabular retroversion. Int Orthop. 2011;35:817–21.
19. Dos Santos-Vaquinhas A, et al. Improvement of surgical time and functional results after do-it-yourself 3D-printed model preoperative planning in acetabular defects Paprosky IIA-IIIB. Orthop Traumatol Surg Res. 2022;108:103277.
20. Reinbacher P, et al. Preoperative templating in THA using a short stem system: precision and accuracy of 2D versus 3D planning method. J Orthop Traumatol. 2022;23:16.
21. Lattanzi R, Viceconti M, Zannoni C, Quadrani P, Toni A. Hip-Op: an innovative software to plan total hip replacement surgery. Med Inform Internet Med. 2002;27:71–83.
22. Watanabe S, et al. Utility of CT-based navigation in revision total hip arthroplasty for a patient with severe posterior pelvic tilt-case report. BMC Musculoskelet Disord. 2020;21:249.
23. Lewinnek GE, Lewis JL, Tarr R, Compere CL, Zimmerman JR. Dislocations after total hip-replacement arthroplasties. J Bone Joint Surg Am. 1978;60:217–20.
24. Sadhu A, et al. Acetabular component position and the risk of dislocation following primary and revision total hip arthroplasty: a matched cohort analysis. J Arthroplast. 2017;32:987–91.
25. Dorr LD, et al. Structural and cellular assessment of bone quality of proximal femur. Bone. 1993;14:231–42.
26. Ellanti P, Mohan K, Moriarity A, Hogan N, McCarthy T. Canal to diaphysis ratio as a risk factor for hip fractures and hip fracture pattern. SICOT J. 2017;3:64.
27. Noble PC, et al. The anatomic basis of femoral component design. Clin Orthop Relat Res. 1988;(235):148–65.
28. Miettinen SSA, et al. Risk factors for intraoperative calcar fracture in cementless total hip arthroplasty. Acta Orthop. 2016;87:113–9.
29. Devane PA, Horne JG. Assessment of polyethylene wear in total hip replacement. Clin Orthop Relat Res. 1999;(369):59–72. https://doi.org/10.1097/00003086-199912000-00007.
30. De Fine M, et al. Is there a role for femoral offset restoration during total hip arthroplasty? A systematic review. Orthop Traumatol Surg Res. 2017;103:349–55.
31. Sakalkale DP, Sharkey PF, Eng K, Hozack WJ, Rothman RH. Effect of femoral component offset on polyethylene wear in total hip arthroplasty. Clin Orthop Relat Res. 2001;(388):125–34. https://doi.org/10.1097/00003086-200107000-00019.
32. Little NJ, Busch CA, Gallagher JA, Rorabeck CH, Bourne RB. Acetabular polyethylene wear and acetabular inclination and femoral offset. Clin Orthop Relat Res. 2009;467:2895–900.
33. Pituckanotai K, et al. Risk of revision and dislocation in single, dual mobility and large femoral head total hip arthroplasty: systematic review and network meta-analysis. Eur J Orthop Surg Traumatol. 2018;28:445–55.
34. Dimitriou D, Tsai T-Y, Kwon Y-M. The effect of femoral neck osteotomy on femoral component position of a primary cementless total hip arthroplasty. Int Orthop. 2015;39:2315–21.

Planning in Robotic-Assisted Total Hip Arthroplasty

10

Sonia K. Chandi, Simarjeet Puri, Colin C. Neitzke, Eytan M. Debbi, and Brian P. Chalmers

10.1 Introduction

Robotic-assisted total hip arthroplasty (THA) was first introduced in the 1990s, with the first robotic THA being performed in 1992 [1]. Over the years, advancements in technology have led to rapid improvements in robotic-assisted THA. Robotic-assisted THA can be classified into two types: haptic/semi-active and autonomous/active. The MAKO robot (Stryker, FL, USA), a semi-active robot requiring surgeon involvement with real-time haptic loop feedback, was FDA-approved for THA in 2010.

The outcomes of THA are influenced by several factors, including surgical approach, patient demographics, and implant design. A major risk factor for poor outcomes, mainly dislocation, implant impingement, wear, and need for revision surgery following THA, is component malpositioning [2–4]. Robotic-assisted systems have the potential to reduce complications and provide more accuracy and precision with component placement [1, 5]. The accuracy of implant placement may contribute to increasing implant survivorship and to lowering rates of revision. Robotic-assisted THA has been associated with lower risks of revision for dislocation, more accurate component positioning, and lower rates of intraoperative complications compared to manual THA [1, 6]. Despite potential advantages of advancements in technology in THA, there are also risks associated with robotic-assisted THA, such as longer operative times and use of additional intraosseous pins, which could contribute to intraoperative complications [1, 6–8]. As the technology continues to improve, further comparative studies are required to determine

S. K. Chandi · S. Puri · C. C. Neitzke ·E. M. Debbi · B. P. Chalmers (✉)
Adult Reconstruction and Joint Replacement Service, Hospital for Special Surgery, New York, NY, USA
e-mail: chalmersb@hss.edu

G. M. Marcheggiani Muccioli et al. (eds.), *Easy Planning in Elective Primary Orthopedic Procedures*, https://doi.org/10.1007/978-3-031-77006-7_10

long-term clinical advantages of robotic-assisted THA. In this chapter, we will review the surgical procedure for robotic-arm-assisted THA using the MAKO robot.

10.2 Surgical Approach

The goal of the surgical approach is to allow for adequate visualization. The MAKO robot has been designed to accommodate multiple approaches in THA including the posterolateral approach, anterolateral approach, and direct anterior approach. Surgical approach is surgeon dependent and determined based on their personal preference and patient characteristics.

10.3 Preoperative Planning

Prior to THA with the MAKO robot, each patient requires a preoperative CT scan of the pelvis and bilateral knees using the MAKO THA CT Scanning Protocol. Once the CT scan has been obtained, the company creates a patient-specific 3D model of the patient's pelvis and femur to allow for preoperative planning of the components. The patient-specific preoperative planning allows for accurate size and positioning of the acetabular cup and femoral stem. Many surgeons also obtain preoperative sitting and standing AP and lateral radiographs of the spine for functional assessment of spinopelvic positioning (Figs. 10.1 and 10.2). This is not required but

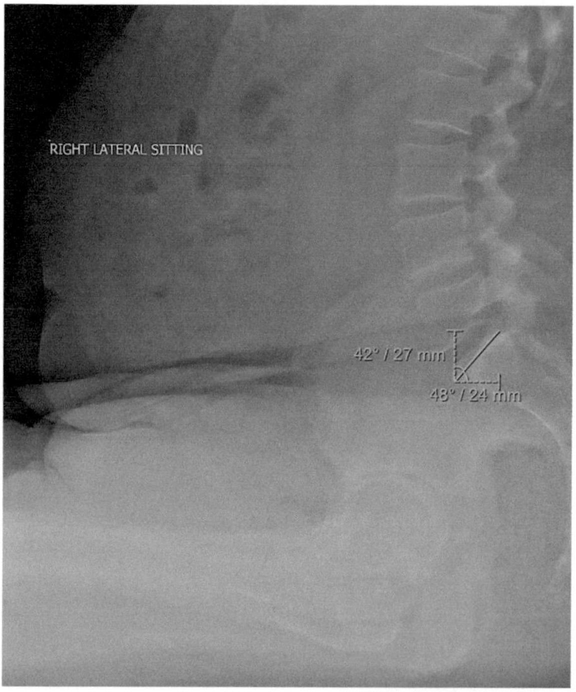

Fig. 10.1 (Left) Sitting lateral radiograph with the sacral slope measured

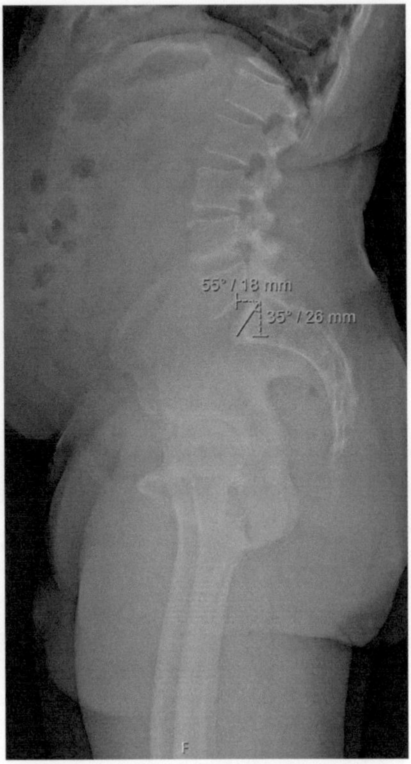

Fig. 10.2 (Right) Standing lateral radiograph with the sacral slope measured

is necessary to utilize the more advanced software that allows preoperative 3D impingement modeling.

In the preoperative planning mode, the surgeon can review hip length and combined offset in comparison to the contralateral hip. The hip length is measured using the landmark of the teardrop of the pelvis and the lesser trochanter (Fig. 10.3). Hip length does not necessarily correlate to leg length and a clinical assessment should be performed along with the computer preoperative planning.

Next, the surgeon can enter the "Cup Plan Mode." In this mode, acetabular cup placement is optimized to achieve desired inclination and version (Fig. 10.4). The cup should be adjusted to ensure good fixation and adequate bony coverage, including being tucked under the anterior wall, so that it is not prominent anteriorly. Using the coronal view, cup size and medialization can be determined (Fig. 10.5). After the acetabular cup is templated, the surgeon can use the "Stem Plan Mode" to plan the femoral stem (Fig. 10.6). In the coronal view, the stem is sized in the distal canal, ensuring the implant is centered in the canal and has good cortical contact. Desired stem offset, version, and head length should be set in this mode. The planned neck cut is established here, and hip length and combined offset values are used to assess how to adjust the implants to achieve desired leg length and offset.

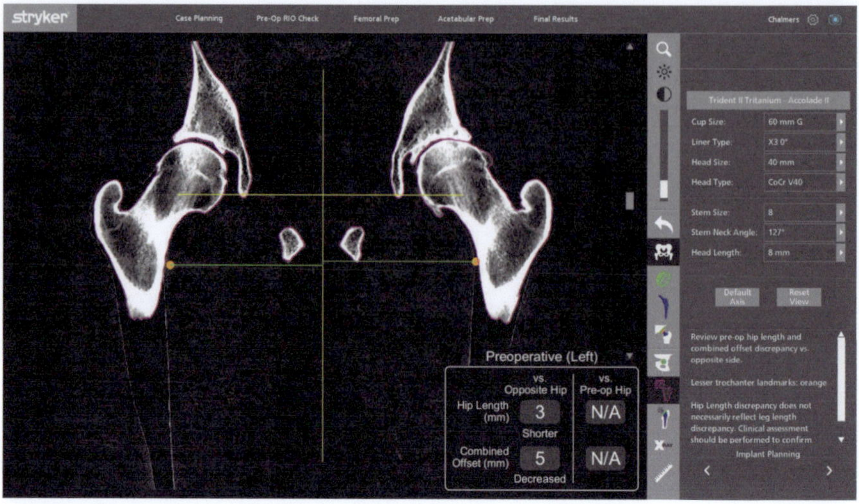

Fig. 10.3 Assessment of preoperative limb length on the planning software

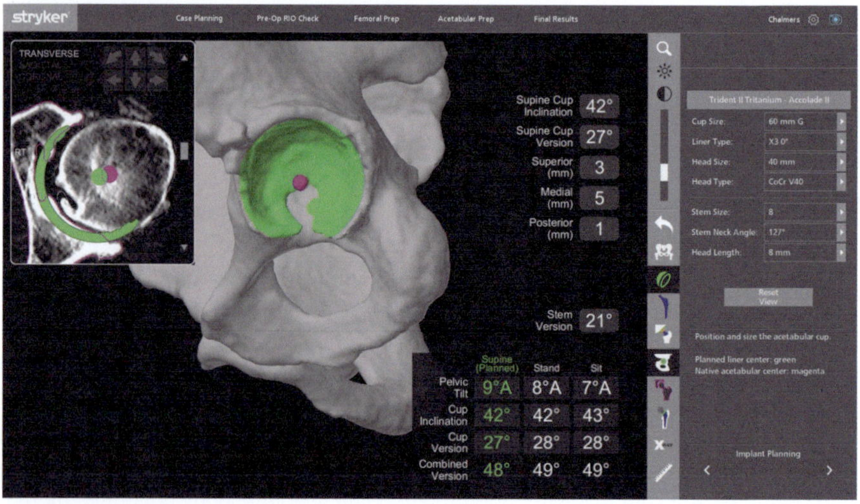

Fig. 10.4 3D planning of the cup size and position

Once the femoral stem, acetabular cup position, and desired articulation (36 head, 40 head, dual mobility, etc.) are templated, the surgeon can perform 3D modeling with range of motion to impingement if preoperative sitting and standing lateral spine radiographs are obtained. On the standing and sitting lateral radiographs, the surgeon should measure the pelvic tilt and sacral slope (Figs. 10.1 and 10.2). These numbers are then entered into the software to allow the software

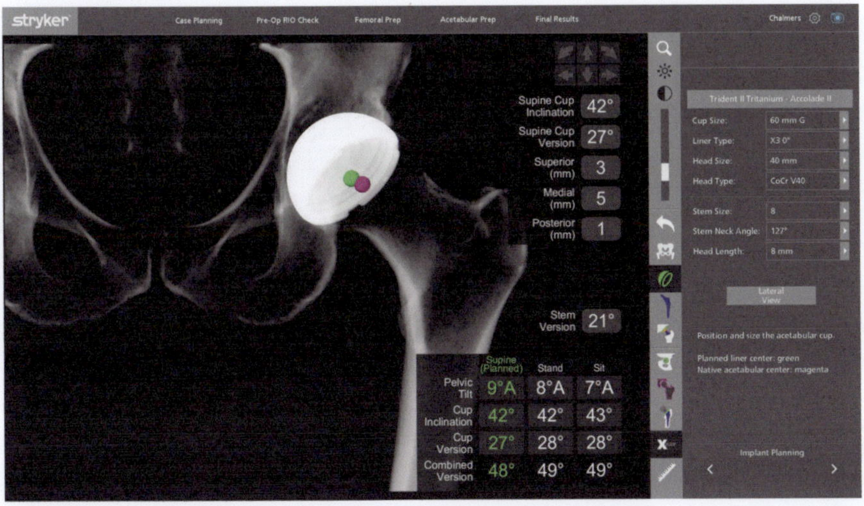

Fig. 10.5 Preoperative simulated radiograph of what the planned acetabular cup will look like on the postoperative radiograph

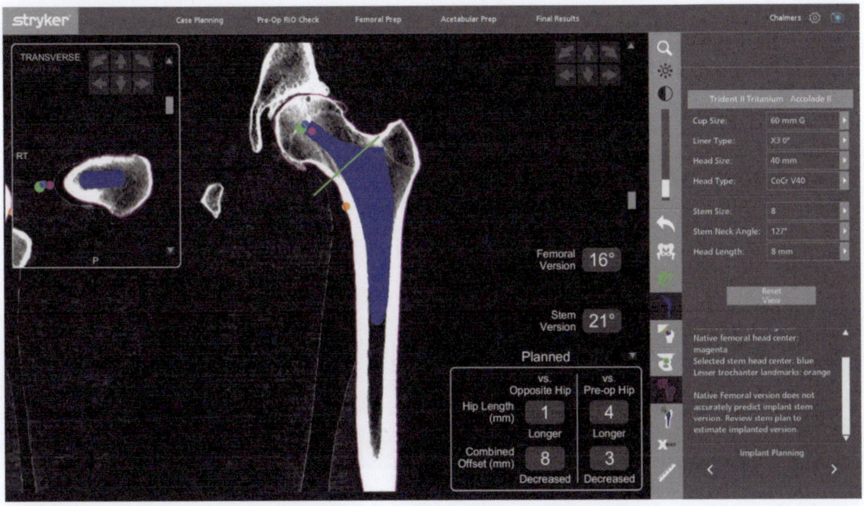

Fig. 10.6 3D planning of the femoral component size, offset, and version

to simulate the pelvic movement in the standing and sitting position to best model impingement for each individual patient. Figure 10.7 shows impingement modeling with the patient standing and the hip in full extension and external rotation; our goal is to achieve 25–30° of external rotation at 10° of extension before any bony or prosthetic impingement. Figure 10.8 shows the hip in 90° of flexion and maximal internal rotation before bony or prosthetic impingement to model the

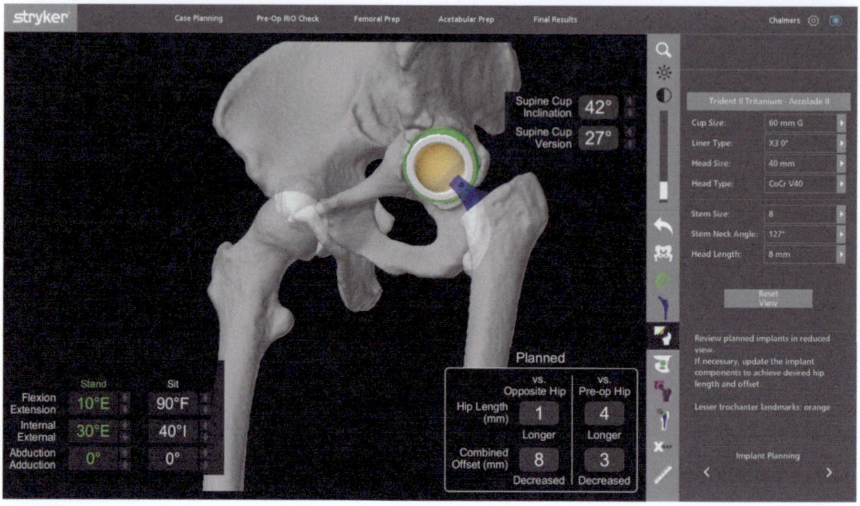

Fig. 10.7 3D impingement modeling in extension and external rotation

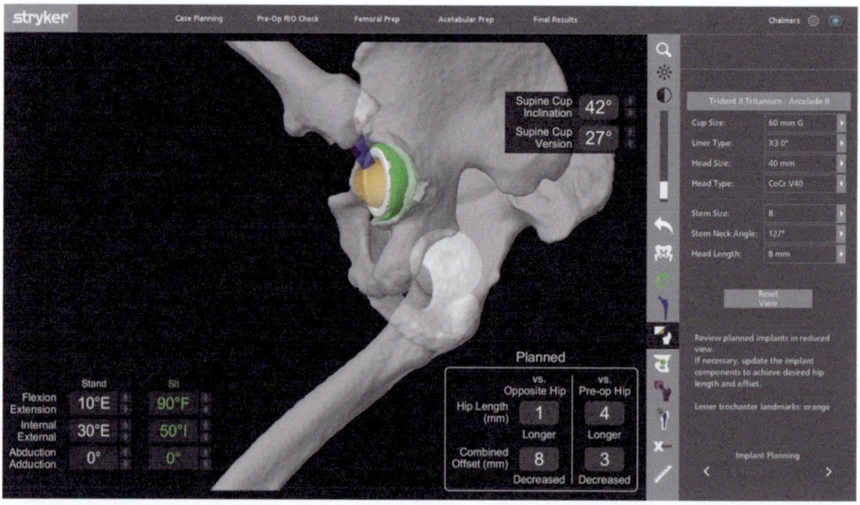

Fig. 10.8 3D impingement modeling in 90° of flexion and maximal internal rotation until bony impingement

patient in the sitting position. Figure 10.9 shows the hip flexing to 120° at 20° of internal rotation to ensure there is no impingement in full flexion. This mode is used to assess if the implant will allow for functional range of motion without impingement. Based on this modeling, the surgeon can adjust cup and stem position to optimize range of motion to impingement. In general, prosthetic impingement can be improved upon by adjusted cup and stem position and femoral and acetabular offset; bony impingement is more difficult to reduce and can be

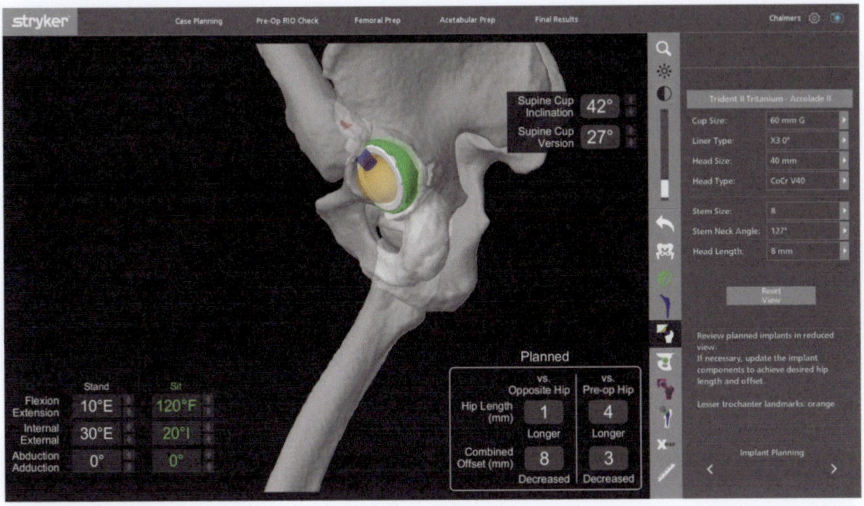

Fig. 10.9 3D templating at 20° of internal rotation to maximal hip flexion prior to bony impingement

improved upon by changing acetabular and femoral offset and femoral anteversion, but less so with changes in cup position.

10.4 Surgical Procedure

After patient positioning, prior to washing and prepping the surgical site, a distal landmark is placed with an EKG lead sticker, which is placed either centered on the patella or slightly inferior to the center of the patella. A Tegaderm is placed on top of the EKG lead sticker to secure it in place. Next, routine sterile prep and drape can be performed.

Once the sterile field is prepped and draped, the pelvic array should be placed. The iliac crest is palpated and a stab incision is made along the lateral aspect of the crest. Using a drill, a pin is placed into the bone on the iliac crest. The three-pin pelvic array clamp is used for alignment of the following two pins. Next, the array adapter is attached to the pelvic array clamp, with the clamp approximately 5 mm above the surface of the skin. The pelvic array is then inserted into the adapter, oriented toward the camera (Fig. 10.10).

The surgical approach can now be performed. After routine exposure, a small checkpoint screw is placed on the bony surface of the greater trochanter and another checkpoint screw is placed about 1 cm above the superior rim of the acetabulum. These checkpoints are used to verify the accuracy of bone registration.

Before the hip is dislocated, the surgeon registers the hip length and offset with the probe in the trochanter checkpoint and the distal EKG lead checkpoint. The hip can then be dislocated. The femoral neck cut can be templated by the software or by

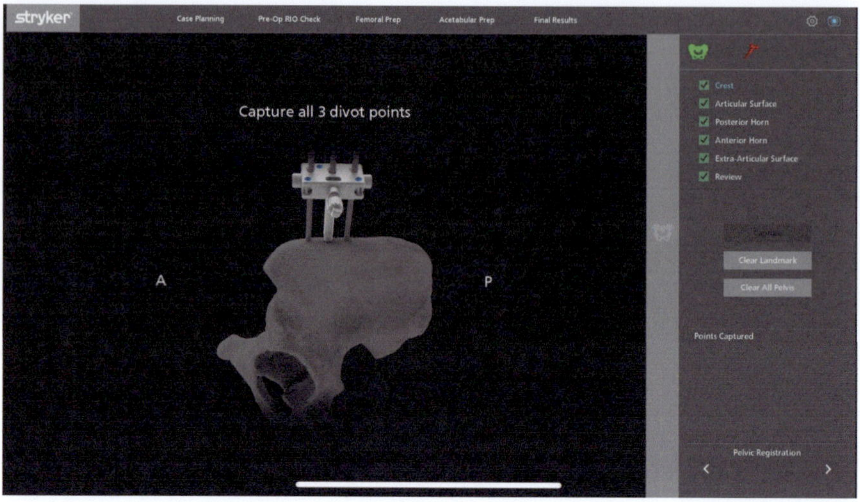

Fig. 10.10 Registering the iliac crest checkpoint

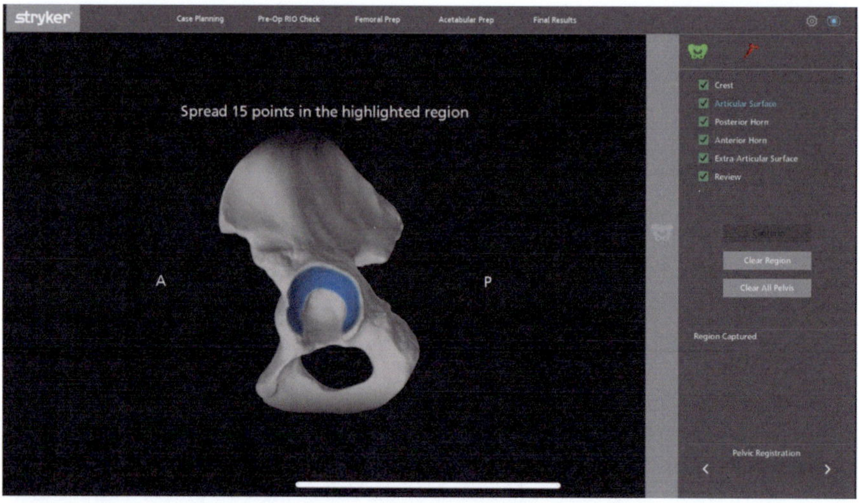

Fig. 10.11 For registration of the bone, 15 points are taken from the intra-articular surface

traditional templating techniques. The femoral neck can be cut as per routine. The femur can then be prepared as per the surgeon's standard routine, keeping in mind the femoral version that was templated on the software.

Once satisfied with femoral implant positioning, the surgeon can prepare the acetabulum. The first step is registration of the acetabulum. The surgeon must capture 15 points in the intra-articular region of the acetabulum (Fig. 10.11) and 15 points in the extra-articular region (Fig. 10.12). The surgeon will also ask you to

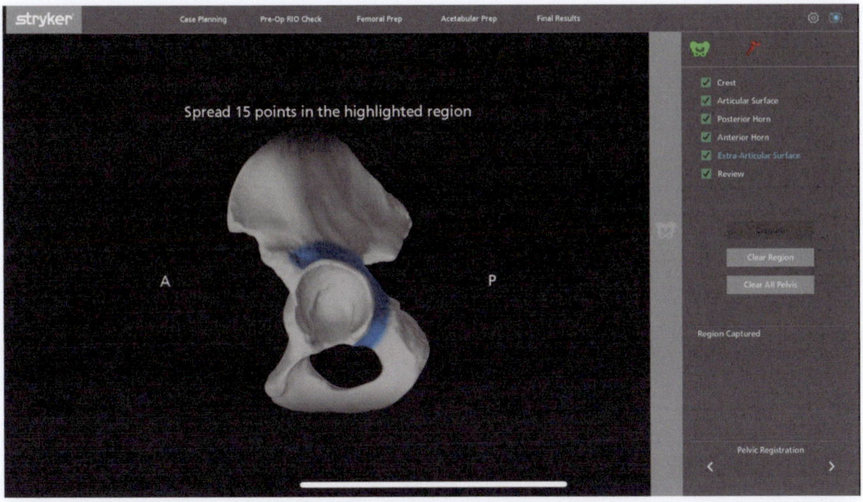

Fig. 10.12 For registration of the bone, 15 points are then taken from the extra-articular surface

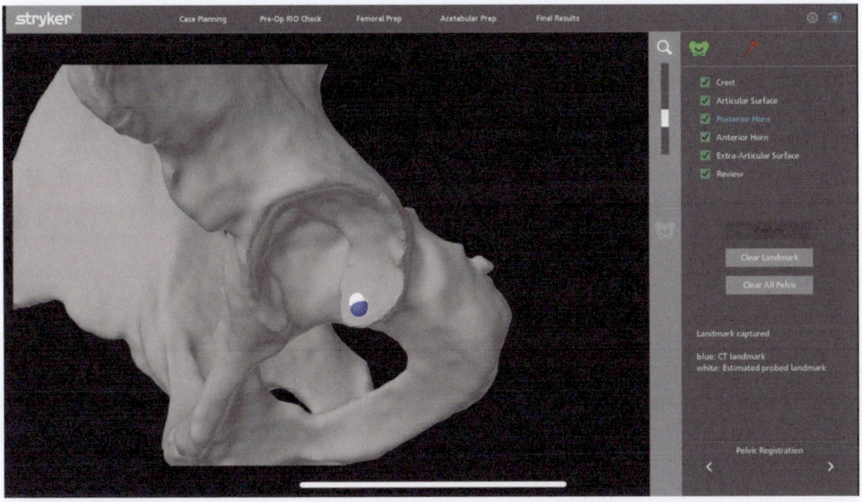

Fig. 10.13 Verification of points on the anterior and posterior horns

identify specific points at the anterior and posterior horns of the acetabulum (Fig. 10.13). Once registration is complete, the surgeon will receive feedback about the accuracy of the registration (Fig. 10.14); additional points or blue spheres may be needed to improve the registration. Following completion of acetabular registration, the surgeon can remove any osteophytes around the acetabular rim. The robotic arm is then brought into the operating field (previously sterile draped) and the surgeon reams the acetabulum using the robotic arm and appropriately sized reamer.

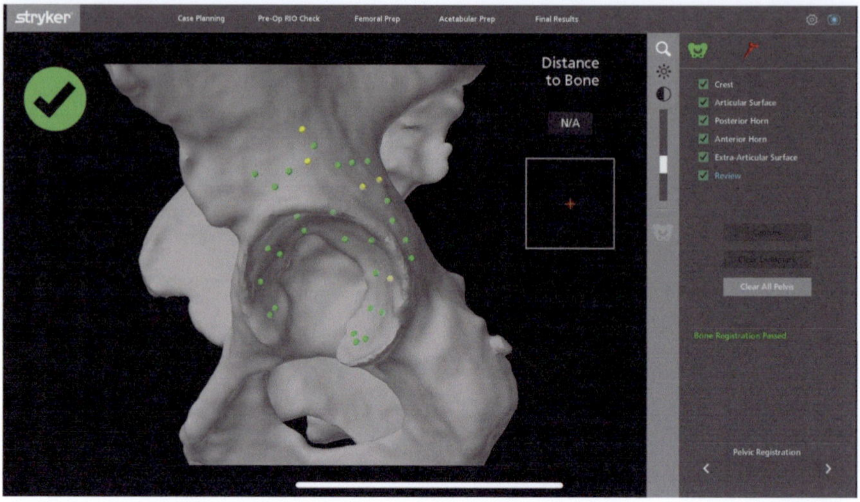

Fig. 10.14 Verification of points registered

The reamer is constrained to the established plan, and the fail-safe stop mechanism will be activated if the reamer exceeds 15° of planned values. The reamer is inserted into the acetabulum and the inclination and anteversion of the reamer handle are adjusted until the preoperative planned values turn green on the screen. The surgeon should then ream until the values representing the cup center of rotation turn green and read as 0 mm. The bone model on the screen displays bone to be reamed in green, which will be removed as the surgeon reams (Fig. 10.4). When only white bone remains on the screen, the reaming has been completed. If the surgeon reams more bone than planned, the area will turn red on the screen. Once acetabular reaming is complete, the final acetabular cup can be placed using the impactor on the robotic arm to maintain accurate version and inclination. The cup is implanted into place by hitting the impactor with a mallet. A probe is used to assess final cup position. Once the cup is fully seated, the robotic arm is removed from the field. Osteophytes can be removed from around the acetabulum and screws can be placed into the cup for additional fixation as desired. The real acetabular liner can then be inserted into the acetabular cup.

The surgeon can then trial with trial femoral heads and the trial broach or elect to place the final stem before trialing. The definitive femoral stem is then manually inserted into the canal. A trial head is placed and the hip is reduced to assess range of motion, stability, leg length, and offset. The probe is utilized on the trochanter and distal EKG lead to ascertain final leg length and offset measurements with the hip reduced during trialing or the final construct (Fig. 10.15).

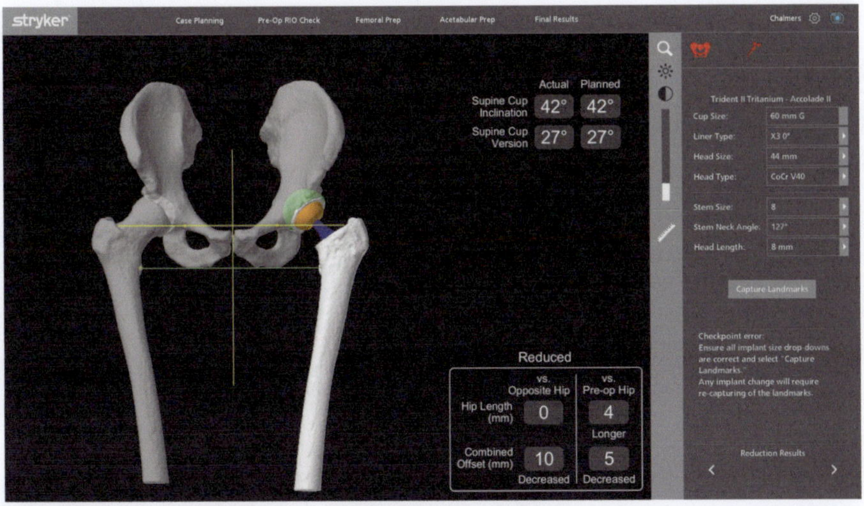

Fig. 10.15 Once the acetabular cup, trial/real femur, and trial head is placed, a trial reduction is performed. The length and offset measurements are captured. All the images are reproduced with permission by Stryker

10.5 Postoperative Management

A postoperative radiograph is obtained to verify implant placement (Fig. 10.16). Postoperative management and rehabilitation for robotic THA is the same as conventional THA and per surgeon's routine.

Take Home Messages

1. Robotic-assisted systems have the potential to reduce complications and provide more accuracy and precision with component placement but longer operative time is required.
2. A patient-specific model is made using the robot-specific CT program.
3. Planning implant positioning also allows a postoperative impingement analysis in order to obtain the best placement possible.
4. Robotic-assisted surgeries allow intraoperative feedback on implant placement, allowing the surgeon follow his planning as accurately as possible.

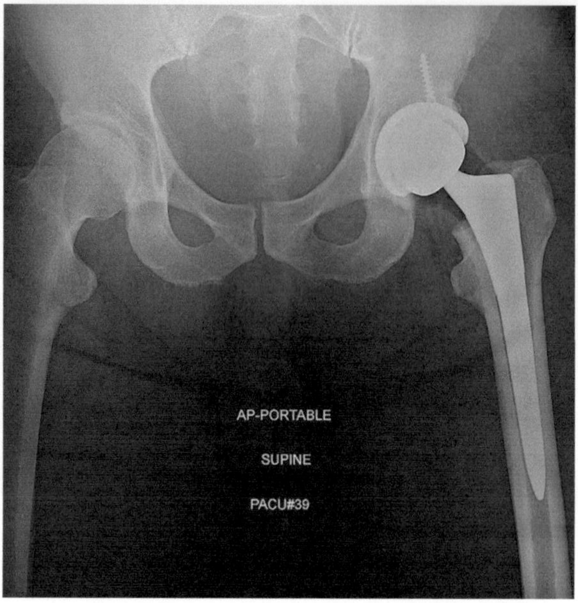

Fig. 10.16 Radiograph taken in the postoperative recovery area

References

1. Chen X, Xiong J, Wang P, Zhu S, Qi W, Peng H, et al. Robotic-assisted compared with conventional total hip arthroplasty: systematic review and meta-analysis. Postgrad Med J. 2018;94:335–41. https://doi.org/10.1136/postgradmedj-2017-135352.
2. Sato K, Sato A, Okuda N, Masaaki M, Koga H. A propensity score-matched comparison between Mako robotic arm-assisted system and conventional technique in total hip arthroplasty for patients with osteoarthritis secondary to developmental dysplasia of the hip. Arch Orthop Trauma Surg. 2022;143(5):2755–61. https://doi.org/10.1007/s00402-022-04524-z.
3. Ando W, Takao M, Hamada H, Uemura K, Sugano N. Comparison of the accuracy of the cup position and orientation in total hip arthroplasty for osteoarthritis secondary to developmental dysplasia of the hip between the Mako robotic arm-assisted system and computed tomography-based navigation. Int Orthop. 2021;45:1719–25. https://doi.org/10.1007/s00264-021-05015-3.
4. Hayashi S, Hashimoto S, Kuroda Y, Nakano N, Matsumoto T, Ishida K, et al. Robotic-arm assisted THA can achieve precise cup positioning in developmental dysplasia of the hip: a case control study. Bone Joint Res. 2021;10:629–38. https://doi.org/10.1302/2046-3758.1010.BJR-2021-0095.R1.
5. Fontalis A, Kayani B, Thompson JW, Plastow R, Haddad FS. Robotic total hip arthroplasty: past, present and future. Orthopaedics and Trauma. 2022;36:6–13. https://doi.org/10.1016/j.mporth.2021.11.002.
6. Bendich I, Vigdorchik JM, Sharma AK, Mayman DJ, Sculco PK, Anderson C, et al. Robotic assistance for posterior approach total hip arthroplasty is associated with lower risk of revision for dislocation when compared to manual techniques. J Arthroplast. 2022;37:1124–9. https://doi.org/10.1016/j.arth.2022.01.085.
7. Sousa PL, Sculco PK, Mayman DJ, Jerabek SA, Ast MP, Chalmers BP. Robots in the operating room during hip and knee arthroplasty. Curr Rev Musculoskelet Med. 2020;13:309–17. https://doi.org/10.1007/s12178-020-09625-z.
8. Kamara E, Berliner ZP, Hepinstall MS, Cooper HJ. Pin site complications associated with computer-assisted navigation in hip and knee arthroplasty. J Arthroplast. 2017;32:2842–6. https://doi.org/10.1016/j.arth.2017.03.073.

Part IV

Osteotomy Around the Hip in Adults

Y. Minoda

11 Planning of Femoral Osteotomy for Hip Dysplasia

Yutaka Inaba, Taro Tezuka, and Yukihide Minoda

11.1 Introduction

Developmental dysplasia of the hip (DDH) includes various changes in hip geometry, from simple dysplasia to complete dislocation of the hip joint. DDH is characterized by pathological changes in the acetabulum and/or femur and associated soft tissue (hip capsule and ligament) abnormalities.

The bony morphological abnormalities in DDH can be divided into two categories. Abnormalities of the acetabulum are typified by a shallow acetabulum, which causes poor coverage of the femoral head by the acetabulum, and morphological abnormalities of the proximal femur are characterized by a more anteverted femoral neck, smaller femoral offset, and narrow medullary canal. Subluxation and dislocation result in the combination of these abnormalities.

In cases of DDH, proximal femoral deformities are mainly coxa valga, excessive anteversion, and narrow canal. Varus osteotomy was introduced by Pauwel for cases of coxa valga in 1950 [1], and the essence of varus osteotomy is to improve mechanical stress by correcting coxa valga. However, varus osteotomy alone rarely improves coverage of the femoral head adequately, and recently most surgeons use pelvic osteotomy, except in special cases such as the completely dislocated hip. In contrast, valgus femoral osteotomy is performed with pelvic osteotomy for Perthes-like deformities or end-stage osteoarthritis due to DDH. This chapter discusses the preoperative planning of varus femoral osteotomy for hips with dysplastic acetabulum and valgus femoral osteotomy for patients with Perthes-like deformities associated with DDH.

Y. Inaba (✉) · T. Tezuka · Y. Minoda
Department of Orthopaedic Surgery, Yokohama City University, Yokohama, Japan
e-mail: yute0131@yokohama-cu.ac.jp

G. M. Marcheggiani Muccioli et al. (eds.), *Easy Planning in Elective Primary Orthopedic Procedures*, https://doi.org/10.1007/978-3-031-77006-7_11

11.2 Radiographic Evaluation

Osteotomies for DDH aim to establish bone stability and prevent arthritis progression. To perform an adequate osteotomy, it is essential to understand the biomechanical principles and bone geometry in each case. Osteotomy of the proximal femur aims not only to change the neck-shaft angle in the coronal plane but also to achieve multiplanar correction, including correction of the anteversion angle and flexion to improve the mechanical environment. For this purpose, radiographic evaluation should be performed using anteroposterior radiography and computed tomography (CT), particularly for anteversion of the femoral neck or anterior acetabular coverage. Abduction and adduction functional views are obtained to evaluate for varus and valgus osteotomy, respectively, to decide the correcting angle. Functional radiographs allow the simulation of virtual postoperative joint congruency and the determination of the correction angle. Osteotomy of the proximal femur changes leg length and femoral offset, which affects leg length discrepancy (LLD) or abduction muscle strength, and surgeons should pay attention to this issue. Excessive de-rotation of the femoral neck is often required in cases with DDH. Preoperative CT imaging is useful for a more detailed characterization of the osseous pathology. If the contralateral side is normal, de-rotation could be planned based on the contralateral anteversion angle of the femoral neck.

11.3 Templating Technique

11.3.1 Varus Femoral Osteotomy

The frequency of varus osteotomy has decreased with the spreading of periacetabular osteotomy. However, it is a necessary surgical technique in special cases such as the case shown in Fig. 11.1, 11.2, 11.3, 11.4, 11.5, and 11.6. Figure 11.1 is the bilateral X-ray image of a 19-year-old woman with severe DDH with a CE angle of −18° in her right hip, classified as Crowe III (Fig. 11.1). The neck-shaft angle showed 148° and the femoral anteversion showed 45°. CT showed 45° of excessive anteversion angle of the femoral neck (Fig. 11.2), and 35° of abduction view showed the improvement of congruency (Fig. 11.3). The periacetabular osteotomy alone could not be sufficient for the improvement of joint congruency; therefore, the combination of varus femoral osteotomy and rotational acetabular osteotomy (RAO) was planned. In this case, RAO and varus femoral osteotomy were planned to achieve an ARO (acetabular roof obliquity) of 0° and AHI (acetabular head index) of 80%. The correction angle of the femoral side was planned to be approximately 20°, taking postoperative leg length discrepancy (LLD) into consideration. The version control in the coronal plane was planned so that femoral anteversion was 20° with reference to the contralateral side. As the operative procedure, 20° of lateral wedge osteotomy using a transtrochanteric approach and de-rotation of the femoral neck was planned to reveal a complete reduction of the hip joint (Fig. 11.4). Figure 11.5 shows the immediate postoperative X-ray image. Figure 11.6 is the

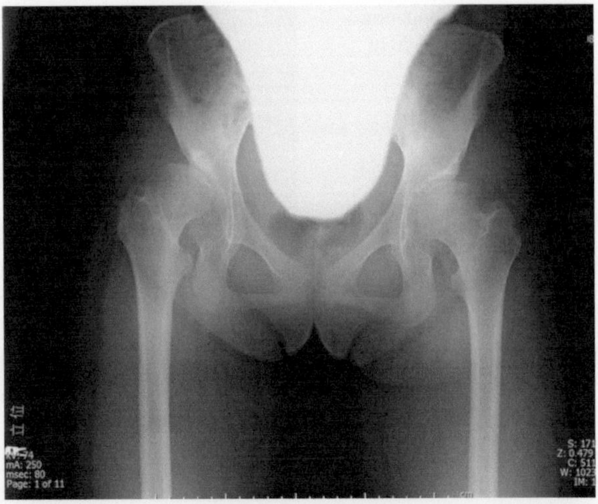

Fig. 11.1 A 19-year-old woman with developmental dysplasia of the hip with subluxation of her left hip classified as Crowe III. She had experienced pain in her left hip 1 year previously

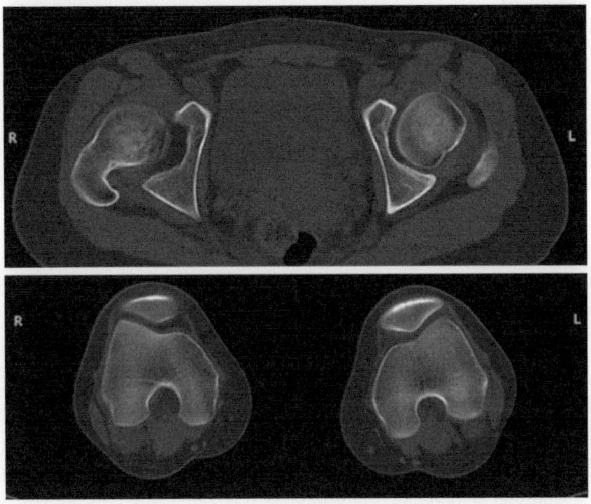

Fig. 11.2 Computed tomography showed excessive femoral anteversion of 45°

X-ray image at 14 years after surgery, and the patient showed no symptoms on her right hip.

11.3.2 Valgus Femoral Osteotomy

Valgus femoral osteotomy is often performed in cases with end-stage hip osteoarthritis showing a femoral head deformity with a capital tear at the medial femoral head or a Perthes-like deformity. The Perthes-like deformity is primarily on the femoral side and can be associated with acetabular dysplasia. Proximal femoral deformity is most notable in the coxa magna, coxa plana, coxa breva, and relative trochanteric overgrowth. In patients with primary femoral deformity, valgus

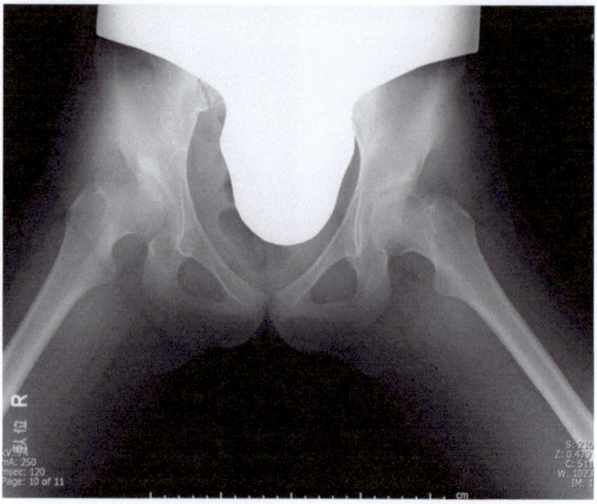

Fig. 11.3 The adduction functional view at 35° of abduction shows improvement in congruency

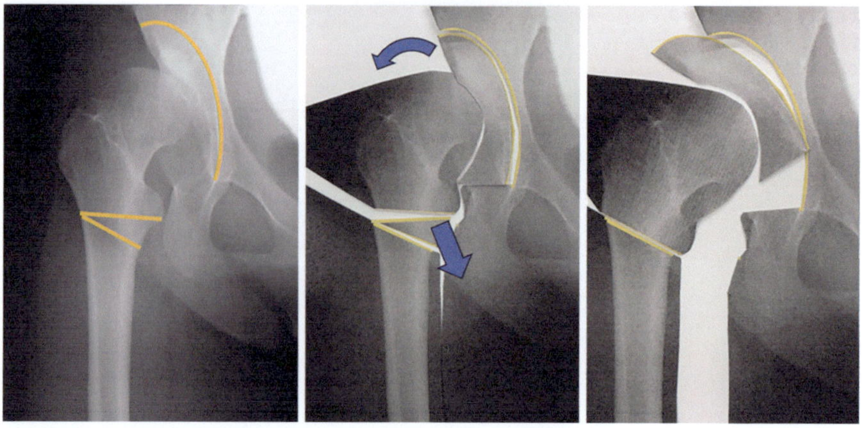

Fig. 11.4 Two-dimensional preoperative planning. The orange lines indicate the osteotomy lines. Rotational acetabular osteotomy (RAO) and varus femoral osteotomy with 20° are planned. The osteotomized wedge bone is removed and the reduction is planned. Preoperative planning of combination of RAO and varus femoral osteotomy

femoral osteotomy with pelvic osteotomy can effectively improve congruency. Preoperative planning is important so that the template for femoral lateral osteotomy is designed to ensure a level joint loading plane, no leg length differences, and prevention of lever arm reduction associated with external rotation to preserve abductor muscle strength. Figure 11.7 shows a 27-year-old woman with DDH and Perthes-like deformity of her left hip, coxa plana, coxa breva, relative trochanteric overgrowth, and 53° excessive anteversion angle of the femoral neck on CT (Fig. 11.8). The adduction functional view at 42° showed the weight-bearing area of

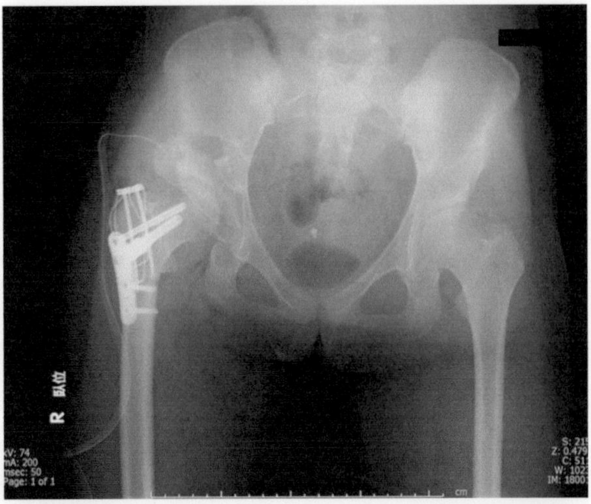

Fig. 11.5 X-ray image just after RAO and femoral varus osteotomy

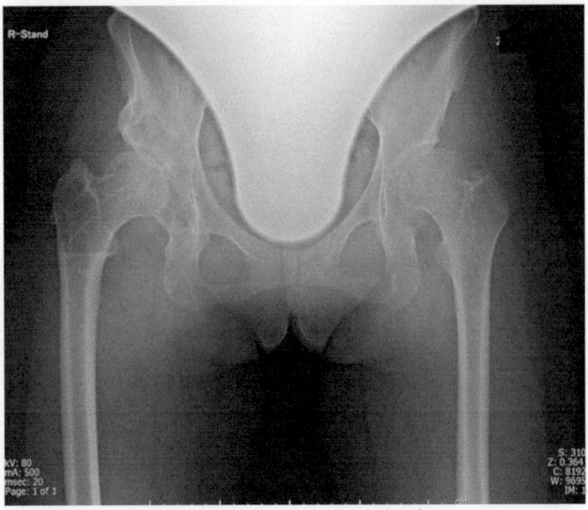

Fig. 11.6 X-ray image at 14 years after surgery. The patient has no symptoms

the femoral head as a horizon (Fig. 11.9). For preoperative planning, 45° of lateral wedge osteotomy using a trans-trochanteric approach and de-rotation of the femoral neck was planned. In addition, lateralization of the femoral shaft was planned to correct LLD (Fig. 11.10). To prevent loss of abductor muscle strength due to a decrease in offset, the greater trochanter was displaced distally and laterally. Figure 11.11 shows an immediate postoperative radiograph. Figure 11.12 shows a radiograph at 13 years after surgery, and the patient showed excellent clinical results. Using this comprehensive approach, both acetabular and femoral deformities can be addressed to optimize hip reconstruction.

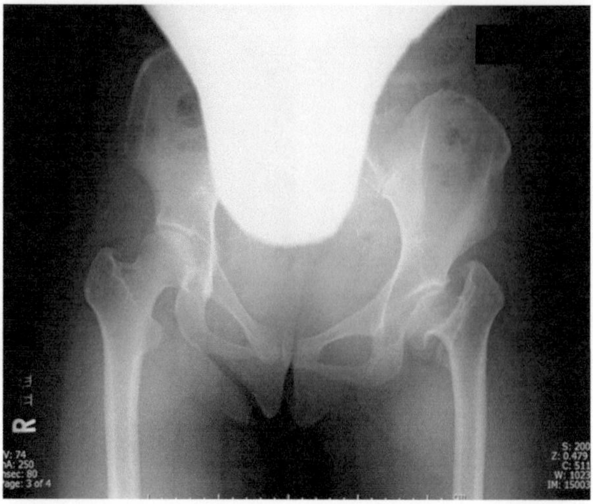

Fig. 11.7 A 27-year-old female with a history of developmental dysplasia of the hip. X-ray shows Perthes-like deformity of the left femoral head, left high-standing greater trochanter, and leg-length discrepancy. She has a 2-year history of progressive left hip pain

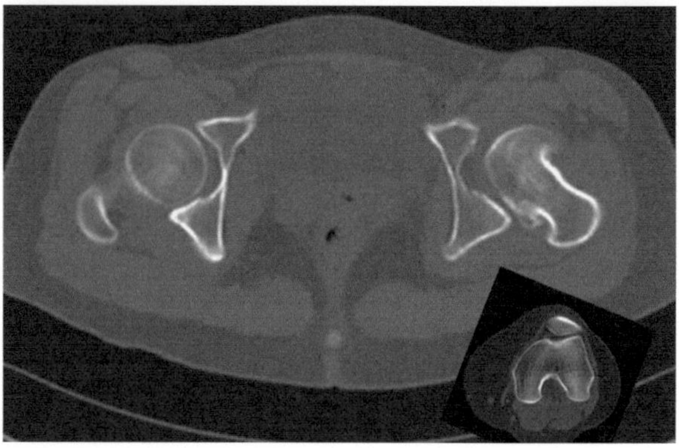

Fig. 11.8 Computed tomography showed excessive femoral anteversion of 53°

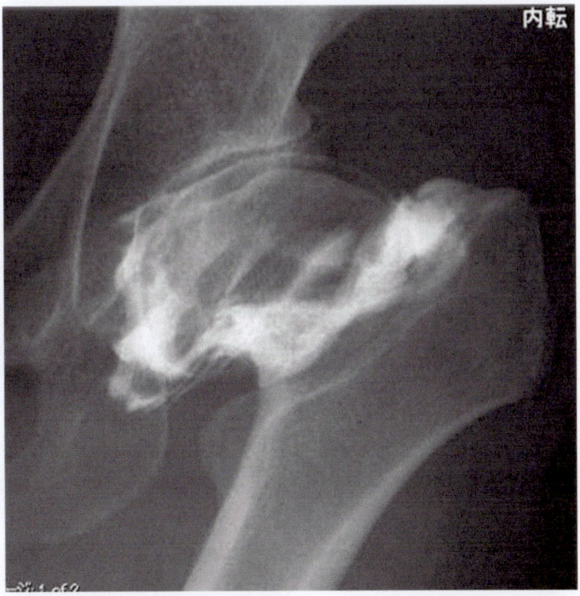

Fig. 11.9 The functional view at 42° of adduction shows the weight-bearing area of the femoral head as horizontal

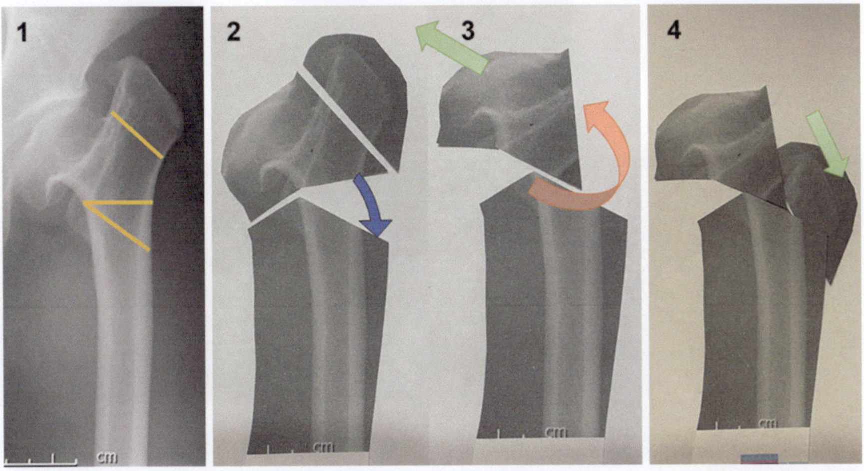

Fig. 11.10 Two-dimensional preoperative planning. The orange lines indicate the osteotomy lines. Valgus corrective angles refer to the radiograph in the functional view. The osteotomized wedge bone is removed and the proximal bone fragment is moved. De-rotation of the femoral neck (orange arrow) and shaft lateralization (green arrow) are planned. Advancement of the greater trochanter laterally and distally is planned (green arrow)

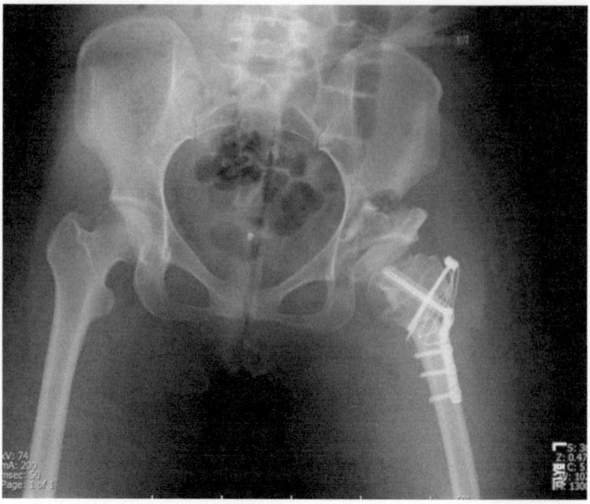

Fig. 11.11 X-ray image just after periacetabular osteotomy and femoral valgus osteotomy shows a lengthened extremity and enhanced congruency of the joint

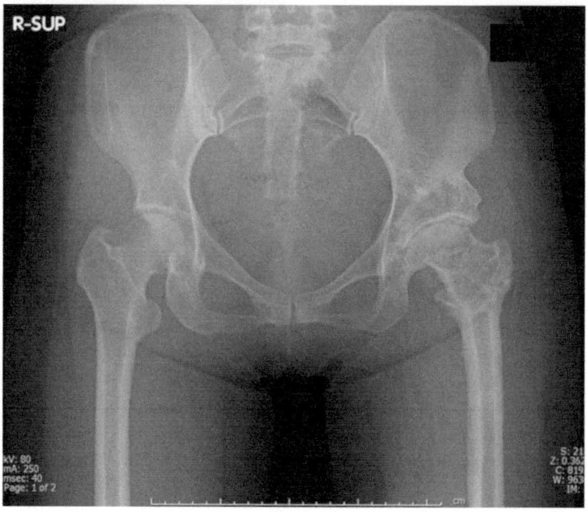

Fig. 11.12 X-ray image at 13 years after surgery. The patient has no symptoms

Take Home Message

1. Severe dysplasia with combined acetabular and femoral deformities is challenging.
2. For preoperative planning, it is important to understand the geometry and mechanical characteristics of the hip joint in each patient.

Reference

1. Pauwels F. [Treatment of coxa valga luxans]. Z Orthop Ihre Grenzgeb. 1950;79:305–15.

Part V

Knee Arthroplasty

G. M. Marcheggiani Muccioli

12 Patient Position and General Setting in Knee Arthroplasty

V. G. Rinaldi, E. Cammisa, I. Sassoli, M. La Verde, A. Fogacci, and Giulio Maria Marcheggiani Muccioli

12.1 Introduction

Optimal patient positioning on the operating table during knee arthroplasty means a safe supine position for the patient without creating an obstacle to the surgeon. All joints should ideally be positioned close to neutral; nerve and skin injuries need to be preserved, and muscles and bony prominence need to be protected by positional aids.

Patient positioning needs to be stable on the operating table, and the surgeon has to spend extra time to ensure that the operating knee can gain the various degrees of flexion needed during surgery and can be easily accessible. Incorrect patient position may result in limited access to the patient's knee during surgery and increase the risk for complications. Limitations and damages during surgery due to the patient's position are unacceptable.

12.2 The Optimal Patient Positioning

The optimal patient positioning for each knee procedure should follow the standard operating procedures (SOPs) [1]. Proper positioning facilitates preoperative skin preparation, appropriate draping, and surgical procedure. Moreover, positioning requires detailed knowledge of anatomy, physiologic principles, and familiarity with the necessary equipment.

The position selected should:

V. G. Rinaldi · E. Cammisa · I. Sassoli · M. La Verde · A. Fogacci ·
G. M. Marcheggiani Muccioli (✉)
2nd Orthopedic and Traumatologic Clinic, IRCCS Istituto Ortopedico Rizzoli, Bologna, Italy
e-mail: giulio.marcheggiani2@unibo.it

G. M. Marcheggiani Muccioli et al. (eds.), *Easy Planning in Elective Primary Orthopedic Procedures*, https://doi.org/10.1007/978-3-031-77006-7_12

- be a correct supine position of the patient close to the operating side of the table;
- provide exposure to the surgical site allowing different flexion positions of the knee without restrictions;
- maintain the patient's comfort and privacy using supports and paddings;
- give access to IV lines and monitoring equipment; and,
- maintain circulation.

The surgeon must find the ideal position for himself during the surgical procedure. A comfortable position means that the surgeon stands or sits without discomfort or pain to prevent early fatigue during the surgery. The table should be placed at an adequate height, which may change during the surgical procedure. The distance difference to the surgeon due to the extension and flexion position of the knee needs to be checked and adjusted before the surgery. Positional aids such as supports and paddings are essential to avoid bony prominence damage and pressure sore, which will occur when external pressure exceeds capillary filling pressure of 32 mmHg [2]. These precautions are even more important for patients with diabetes mellitus, poor vascularization, elderly age, or low body mass index with an increased risk for pressure ulcers [3]. Moreover, all bony prominences need to be well-protected and padded. Nerves may be inadvertently injured during surgery due to pressure or abnormal joint position [4].

There are different options for patient positioning on the operating table. However, patients need to be supine for a knee arthroplasty procedure (Fig. 12.1). The head and the spine need to be aligned and the neck in a neutral position; the shoulders should not be abducted to more than 90°, and the elbow should be flexed to less than 90°. Moreover, the forearm should be positioned in a neutral or slightly supinated position. This setting helps to avoid ulnar nerve compression, which is the most frequent site of perioperative neuropathy [5].

Lateral support at the level of the tight and foot support will help the assistant to keep the knee in an adjustable flexed position (Figs. 12.2 and 12.3). Usually, total knee replacement is performed from 70° to 120° of knee flexion. It is mandatory

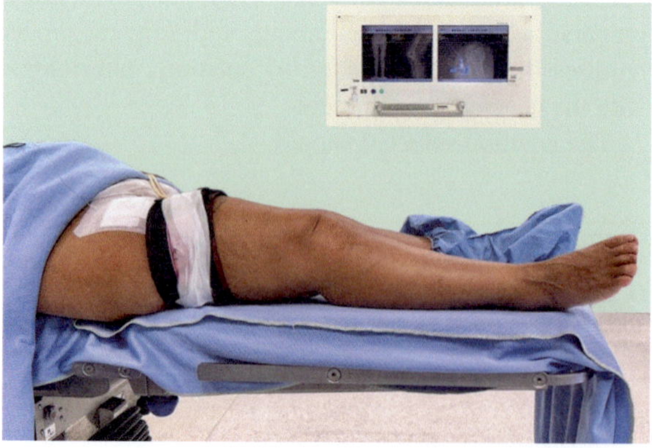

Fig. 12.1 Patient needs to be positioned supine for knee arthroplasty procedures

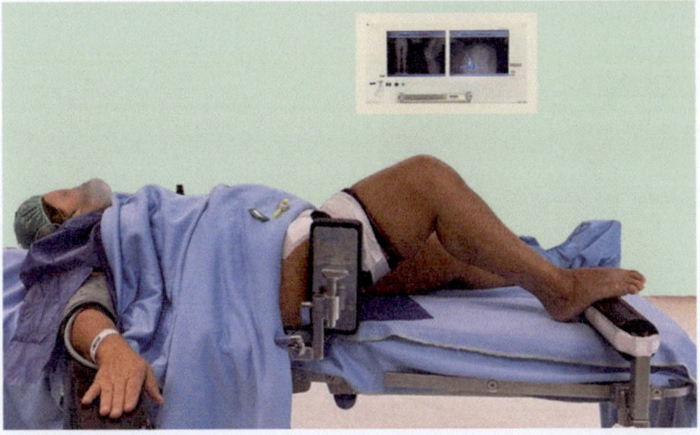

Fig. 12.2 The head and the spine need to be aligned and the neck in a neutral position; the shoulders should not be abducted to more than 90°, and the elbow should be flexed to less than 90°. Special attention is paid to protecting bony prominence sites. The lower limb can be positioned using tight and foot supports. The support at the thigh is used to avoid external rotation of the hip. The foot support keeps the knee in an adequate position

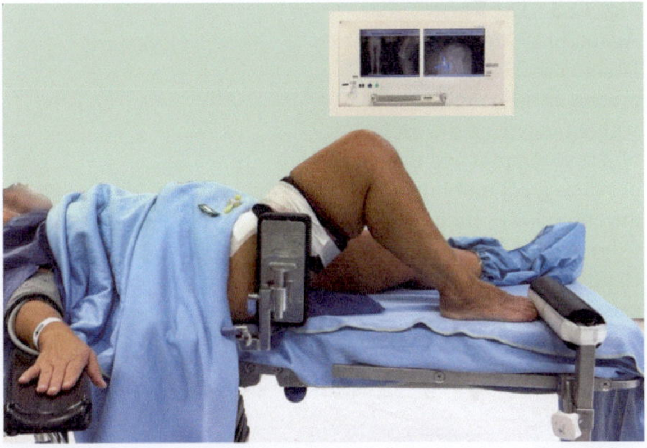

Fig. 12.3 With the assistance of foot support, knee flexion can be adjusted according to the surgeon's needs

that the knee can easily be positioned from flexion to extension and vice versa. Foot support location is essential to set the knee joint degree of flexion.

The use of a sterile pad may allow the required degrees of flexion to be gained to perform the tibial cut (Fig. 12.4a and b). Holding the knee too flexed can be counterproductive as it results in collateral ligaments and extensor apparatus tightening; thus, more force is needed surrounding soft tissues.

Moreover, another possible solution is to use a hydraulic leg holder that can allow free flexion and extension of the knee without manual assistant help. Another option may be using a knee positioner that can provide excellent stability and an ample range of motion. Furthermore, as it does not require lateral support, it could be helpful when carrying out robotic or navigated surgery (Fig. 12.5).

The use of tourniquets in knee arthroplasty is a debated topic [6–9]. Many surgeons prefer to carry out knee replacement surgery with the aid of a tourniquet, which has potential benefits, including limiting blood loss during surgery and

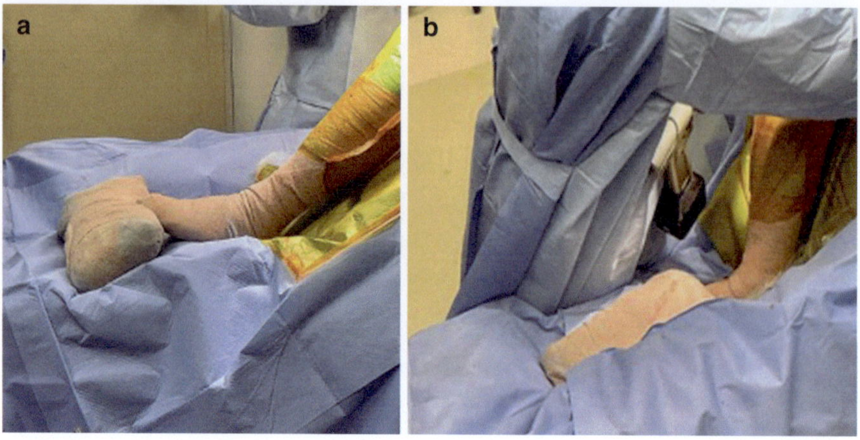

Fig. 12.4 (**a, b**) The use of a sterile pad can help the surgeon to achieve deep flexion when it is needed

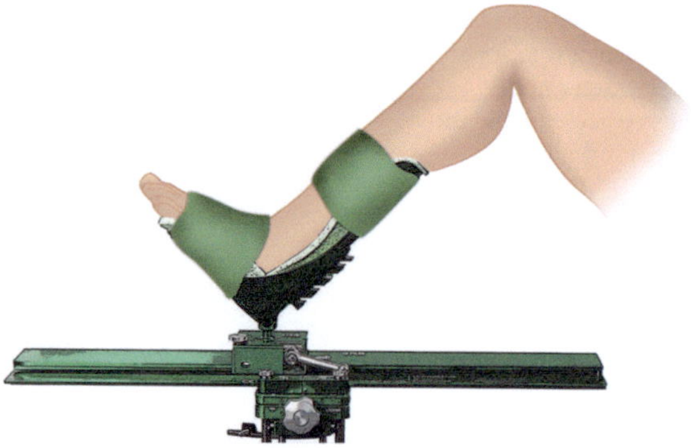

Fig. 12.5 The Mayo Adapt2Fit® Modular Knee Positioner allows for precise ROM control without requiring the use of lateral support and thus provides great mobility of the entire lower limb.

making it easier to conduct the operation [9]. However, tourniquet use may increase the risk of pain and complications for patients in the early rehabilitation program [7].

If a tourniquet is used during surgery, the cuff should be positioned as proximal as possible on the thigh to consent to free access to the knee. Additionally, it is important to ensure that the tourniquet cuff is chosen to match the limb size and shape at the desired cuff location. It is crucial to pay close attention to the positioning of the tourniquet cuff to avoid struggles in knee exposure and patella eversion.

In conclusion, the safe positioning of the patient for surgery in the operating room is the surgeon's responsibility. Furthermore, the surgeon should always perform a final check of the patient's position before disinfection and sterile draping start.

Take Home Messages

1. Patient positioning is crucial for a successful total knee replacement surgery.

2. Positioning requires detailed knowledge of anatomy, physiologic principles, and familiarity with the necessary equipment.
3. All the bony prominences should be well-protected and padded.
4. Knee should be positioned to allow free flexion to extension range of motion and vice versa, and foot support location is essential to set the knee joint degree of flexion during surgery.
5. Incorrect position of the patient may result in limited access to the patient's knee during surgery and will increase the risk of complications.
6. Safe positioning of the patient for surgery in the operating room is the surgeon's responsibility.

References

1. Bleyl JU, Heller AR. [Standard operating procedures and operating room management: improvement of patient safety and the efficiency of processes]. Wien Med Wochenschr. 2008;158:595–602.
2. Lyder CH, Ayello EA. Pressure ulcers: a patient safety issue. In: Hughes RG, editor. Patient safety and quality: an evidence-based handbook. Rockville, MD: Agency for Healthcare Research and Quality; 2008.
3. Liang M, Chen Q, Zhang Y, He L, Wang J, Cai Y, Li L. Impact of diabetes on the risk of bedsore in patients undergoing surgery: an updated quantitative analysis of cohort studies. Oncotarget. 2016;8:14516–24.
4. Bage T, Power DM. Iatrogenic peripheral nerve injury: a guide to management for the orthopaedic limb surgeon. EFORT Open Rev. 2021;6:607–17.
5. Prielipp RC, Morell RC, Walker FO, Santos CC, Bennett J, Butterworth J. Ulnar nerve pressure: influence of arm position and relationship to somatosensory evoked potentials. Anesthesiology. 1999;91:345–54.
6. Arthur JR, Spangehl MJ. Tourniquet use in total knee arthroplasty. J Knee Surg. 2019;32:719–29.
7. Ayik O, Demirel M, Birisik F, Ersen A, Balci HI, Sahinkaya T, Batibay SG, Ozturk I. The effects of tourniquet application in total knee arthroplasty on the recovery of thigh muscle strength and clinical outcomes. J Knee Surg. 2021;34:1057–63.
8. Wu Y, Lu X, Ma Y, Zeng Y, Xiong H, Bao X, Shen B. Efficacy and safety of limb position on blood loss and range of motion after total knee arthroplasty without tourniquet: a randomized clinical trial. Int J Surg Lond Engl. 2018;60:182–7.
9. Zhang W, Li N, Chen S, Tan Y, Al-Aidaros M, Chen L. The effects of a tourniquet used in total knee arthroplasty: a meta-analysis. J Orthop Surg. 2014;9:13.

Planning in Unicompartmental (Medial, Lateral, and Patellofemoral) Knee Artroplasty

13

S. Fratini, I. Sassoli, A. Fogacci, M. P. Neri, M. Lo Presti, and Giulio Maria Marcheggiani Muccioli

13.1 Introduction

Differently from total knee arthroplasty (TKA), which can, at least to a certain attempt, correct the deformity and the joint line, unicompartmental knee replacement (UKA) is mainly a resurfacing act.

In the quest for the minimal and longer-lasting implant possible, this option has become more and more appealing, especially with the advent of robotic assistance, allowing the surgeon for an almost-perfect positioning with respect to the planning [1].

The main focus for the surgeon in this pursuit of precision should be implant survival. The drawback of improper positioning is an equally improper force balance, therefore leading to either stress or wear, with an increased failure risk.

The first part of the planning is patient selection in order to provide higher chances both for quality of life and implant survival and the best treatment possible. Nowadays, the usual topics on which the scientific community debates are age, weight, deformity, and stability.

Those—once strict—criteria, nowadays, are much more lenient, given the improvement in implant placement, materials, and overall survivorship. Of course, the surgeon should remember that great obesity, deformity larger than 15°, and instability are still red flags to be aware of [2, 3].

S. Fratini · I. Sassoli · A. Fogacci · M. P. Neri · M. Lo Presti
G. M. Marcheggiani Muccioli (✉)
2nd Orthopedic and Traumatologic Clinic, IRCCS Istituto Ortopedico Rizzoli, Bologna, Italy
e-mail: giulio.marcheggiani2@unibo.it

G. M. Marcheggiani Muccioli et al. (eds.), *Easy Planning in Elective Primary Orthopedic Procedures*, https://doi.org/10.1007/978-3-031-77006-7_13

13.2 Radiographic Examination

Radiographic examination is key and should be performed before any partial knee arthroplasty to assess the deformity and the axis of the lower limbs and the osteoarthritis (OA) grade.

The usual series of radiographical studies for pre-operatory knee evaluation includes a long-standing view of the knee for axis evaluation and contralateral comparison, lateral plain radiographs, and skyline views. The latter is essential for patellofemoral replacement but is not performed routinary in every hospital (see Fig. 14.3, Chap. 14).

As per total knee replacement, a long-standing view of the knee allows to draw both femoral and tibial anatomical and mechanical axes, the difference between them, namely the anatomical mechanical angle (AMA), the hip-knee-ankle (HKA) angle, and the Paley's angles, such as mechanical medial proximal tibial angle (mMPTA), mechanical lateral distal femoral angle (mLDFA), and joint line convergence angle (JLCA), which are key for a complete analysis of the deformity (Fig. 13.1).

Evaluation of any extraarticular deformity must be evaluated as well to check the joint line, which could be altered if the deformity is close to the joint line itself. The

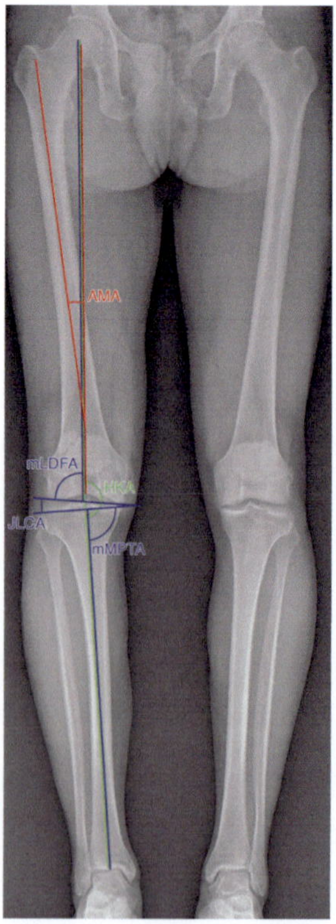

Fig. 13.1 Frontal knee angles (long-standing projection)

goal for UKA is to perform a resurfacing of the compartment, giving the knee the surface that was originally present in the pre-osteoarthritic state.

Posterior tibial slope (PTS) is the single-most important evaluation to be done in lateral radiographs, closely followed by patellar height, femoral offset, and the presence of osteophytes. Those latter measures are more important in the case of a total knee replacement because they can be greatly affected by the implant positioning, but they need to be considered on UKAs as well. Regarding PTS, there is no consensus regarding its calculation method. A valid compromise is obtained by subtracting the angle between the tangent to the tibial medial condyle and the long axis of the tibia to 90°. The long axis of the tibia is determined by drawing a line passing through the center of two circles: one midway between the anterior and posterior border of the tibia at the level of the tibial tubercle and the other 5 cm distal to the tubercle (Fig. 13.2) [4–6].

Lastly, skyline radiographs display the patellofemoral joint, allowing measurement of the patellar tilt angle, shift, and sulcus angle.

Almost every knee replacement manufacturer provides templates for their implants, which can be useful in programming the sizing and placement of the implant. Alternatively, the surgeon can rely on templating programs like OrthoView™, which can interface with PACS and provide precise templating for

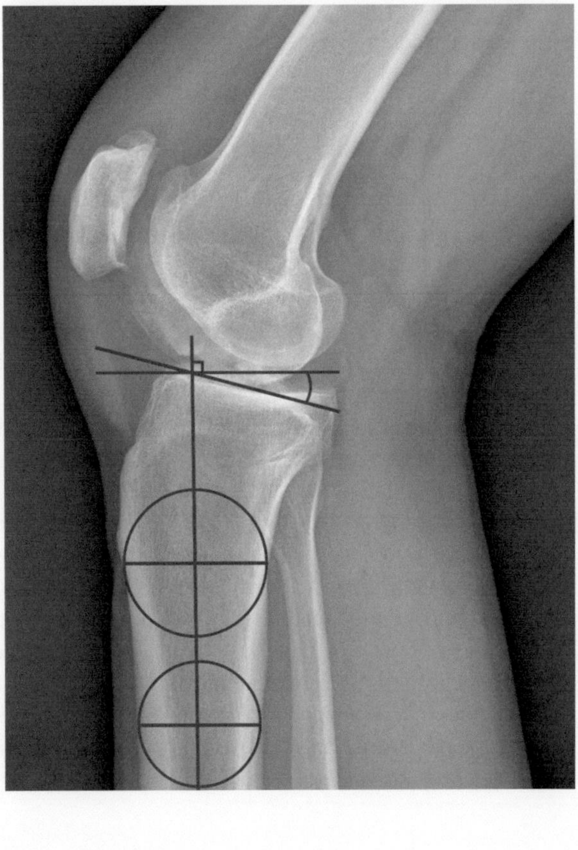

Fig. 13.2 Tibial slope (lateral projection)

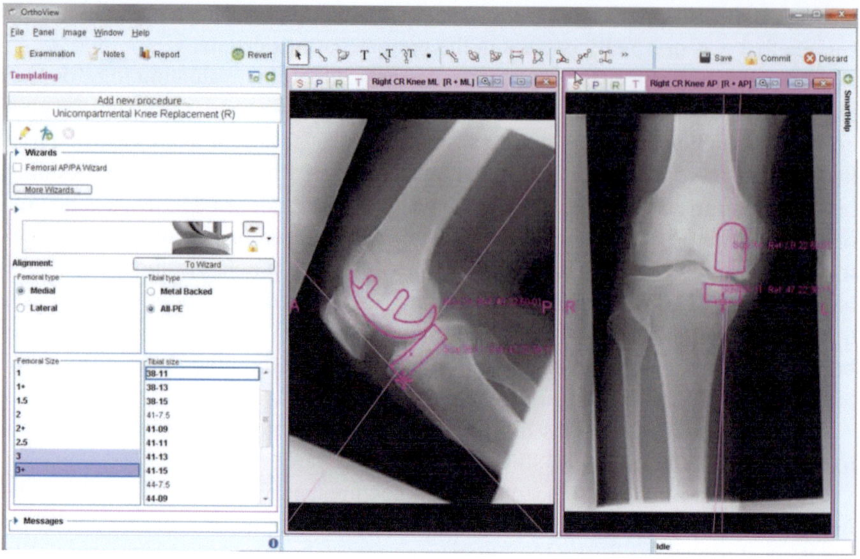

Fig. 13.3 OrthoView™ planning example. Reproduced with permission by Materialise OrthoView™ (Southampton, UK)

each implant included in the database (Fig. 13.3). The images must be calibrated to avoid magnification errors. This is usually achieved by placing a radiopaque marker of known size, such as a 32 mm hip replacement head prosthesis, within the X-ray field of view (see Fig. 14.3, Chap. 14).

13.3 Digital Planning in Medial Unicompartmental Knee Arthroplasty

Medial UKAs are circa 90% of every unicompartmental knee replacement.

Most recent inclusion criteria for medial UKA include advanced medial compartment osteoarthritis or osteonecrosis, functional anterior cruciate ligament (ACL), which can be reconstructed in selected cases together with the prosthesis, preservation of the lateral compartment, correctible varus deformity <10°, flexion deformity <15°, and patient age of between 18 and 80 years [7].

Factors considered as contraindications some years ago, such as young age, high level of activity, obesity, presence of lateral osteophytes, chondrocalcinosis, and low-grade patellofemoral arthritis, are not nowadays considered absolute contraindications anymore. Inflammatory arthritis, hemochromatosis, hemophilia, multicompartment disease, immobility, or any other neurological condition are, on the other hand, still absolute contraindications.

When planning a medial UKA, it is first important to have great confidence and knowledge of the implant used, as different manufacturers can use different references to allow correct cuts.

The amount of proximal tibial cut is crucial because adequate resection is key to obtaining the proper space during flexion. It is crucial to evaluate the flexion space after the tibial proximal cut to obtain a proper extension space after femoral osteotomies. Always keep in mind that every step and cut is linked to the next one.

Tibial cuts are the foundation of medial UKAs: the amount of osteotomy reflects on the tibial axis and should be kept at a minimum. Ideally, the surgeon should always use the minimum insert available.

The main parameters to be evaluated are the direction of the cut and resection depth. Ideally, the cut direction should allow for an overall 3° varus anatomical axis, or the cut can be performed perpendicularly to the tibial mechanical axis to protect the femoral component by the adduction momentum. Whatever choice the surgeon makes, it is crucial to (1) avoid overcorrection and (2) cut the minimal depth possible in order to restore the pre-osteoarthritic alignment.

The sagittal cut should preserve the ACL fibers. Make sure to avoid any posterior overhang of the tibial component (Fig. 13.4).

The femoral cut, then, has to be performed. Some implants will have a guide dependent on the tibial cut, while others allow for further modifications. The component must be well positioned frontally and rotationally, according to the planning previously made (Fig. 13.5). Mediolateral positioning is generally obtained and

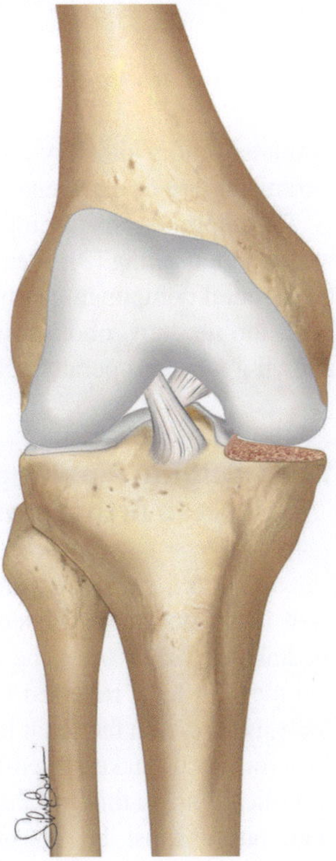

Fig. 13.4 Tibial cut, frontal view, note the sagittal cut just next to ACL fibers. Copyright of Silvia Bassini, 2024. All rights reserved

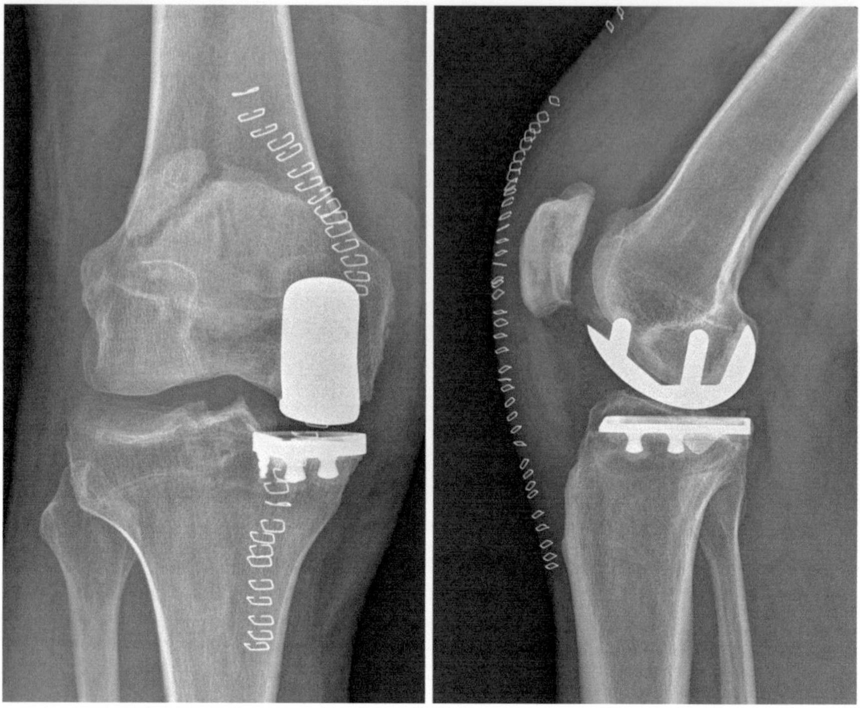

Fig. 13.5 Medial unicompartmental knee replacement

evaluated under direct view, while varus–valgus alignment can be assessed via intramedullary or extramedullary reference, depending on the implant.

The improper positioning of the femoral component is a frequent cause of early wear and loosening [8]. Ideally, the points of contact between the polyethylene and the femoral component should lay on the rotational center of the component itself. With the modern robotic-assisted approaches, this can be seen prior to the cuts, allowing for intraoperative check and postimplant confirmation (see Chap. 15).

13.4 Digital Planning in Lateral Unicompartmental Knee Arthroplasty

Lateral UKA is performed circa 10 times less frequently than its medial counterpart, even if isolated lateral osteoarthritis is not that much less frequent (25% for the medial side vs. 10% for the lateral side). This is mainly due to surgeon preference and the skill level required for satisfactory and constant positioning. Recent meta-analysis shows, in fact, that lateral UKA shows an overall survivorship of more than 98% for metal-backed fixed-bearing implants [9, 10].

Indications, in this case, are mostly superimposable with the ones for the medial side, but it must be considered the frequent association of lateral OA with inflammatory diseases, genu valgum, and patellofemoral OA, especially in long-standing women. In those patients, the mechanical axis passes through the lateral side of the knee, concurring to increase the risk of patellar maltracking and/or hyperpression. Passive ligamentous correctability in case of a valgus deformity is key. In case of a fixed deformity, the surgeon should prefer a TKA for better ligament balancing.

From a planning point of view, lateral UKA cannot be the reflection of the positioning of a medial UKA as the lateral compartment has different anatomy and biomechanics with respect to the medial side of the knee. The femoral condyles are asymmetric, and the lateral one has an increased curvature radius posteriorly, with a slightly longer anteroposterior axis and it is wider at the center of the intercondylar notch. The lateral tibial plateau protrudes circa 3–4 mm more lateral than the medial one and this can lead to place the tibial component too laterally.

The tibial cut should be performed considering a minimal resection (max 5 mm, usually the goal should be 2–4 mm) because the cartilage defect is usually more on the femoral side. The transverse osteotomy should be perpendicular to the mechanical tibial axis, with a neutral anteroposterior slope (0° with respect to the native slope).

The sagittal tibial cut is key: it should be performed between the most medial part of the lateral plateau posteriorly to the ACL insertion when in flexion and the most medial part of the tibial plateau anteriorly to the ACL insertion when in extension (Fig. 13.6).

The femoral cut should be calculated on the long-standing view on the X-ray to provide an accurate plane with the full bearing on the knee. Usually, the target for the distal femoral cut is 3–6° valgus.

The rotation of the femoral component is equally (if not more) important because the lateral femoral condyle diverges compared to the medial side. Moreover, accounting for the "screw-home" mechanism, the tibia externally rotates between 0° and 20°, tightening the ACL and locking the knee. The surgeon has to find the best compromise between an anatomically centered position with respect to the

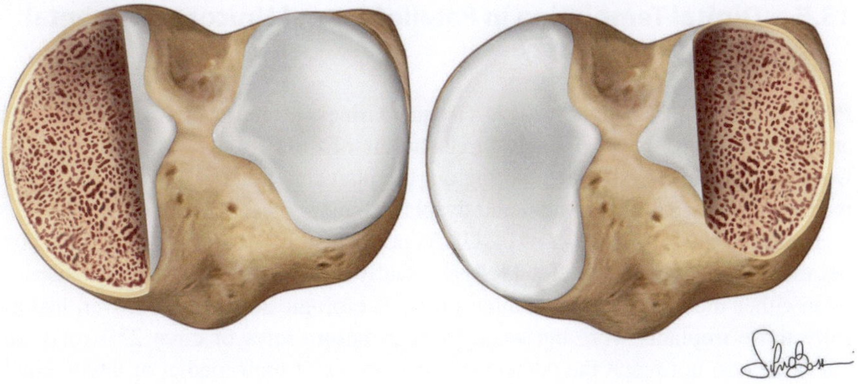

Fig. 13.6 Sagittal cuts, medially and laterally.

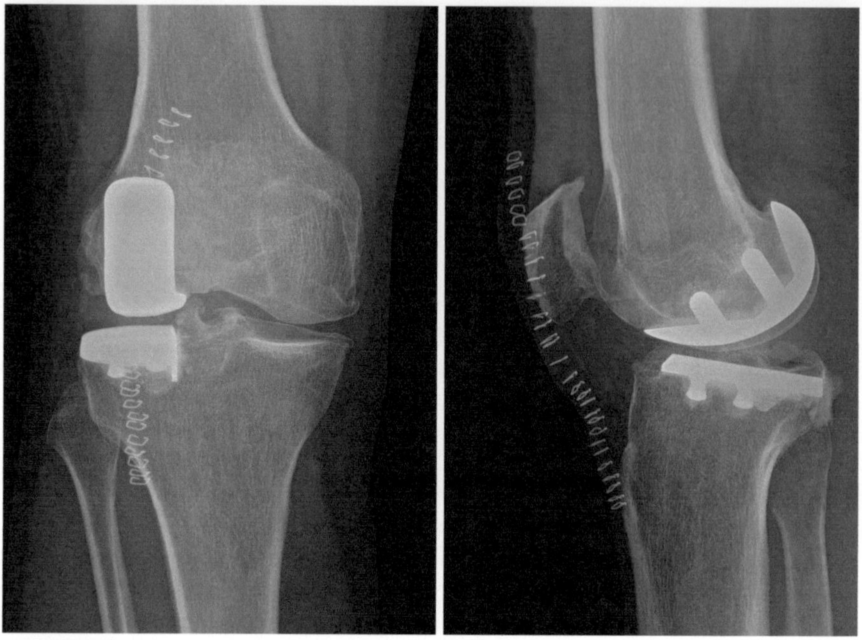

Fig. 13.7 Lateral unicompartmental knee replacement

lateral femoral condyle and a long axis that is perpendicular to the tibial plateau. A "perfect" (which is not!) placement in flexion will inevitably lead to an excessive internal rotation in extension and impingement on the tibial spine. To avoid this, the femoral component should be never oversized and positioned as lateral as possible on the femoral condyle, without removing lateral osteophytes. As per the medial side, never overcorrect (Fig. 13.7).

13.5 Digital Templating in Patellofemoral Unicompartmental Knee Arthroplasty

Patellofemoral (PF) osteoarthritis is a frequent illness affecting up to 20% of women and 10% of men. Approximately three-fourths of the PF UKAs are performed in women, with several studies pointing out the plausible association with the higher incidence of knee malalignment and dysplasia.

However, the total number of PF UKAs performed is circa 1% of all UKAs, both because surgeons tend to prefer TKA, especially if there is already mild osteoarthritis in either medial or lateral compartment, or biologic surgery. Moreover, historically those implants were burdened by high failure rates of circa 25%, and still today they do not reach the percentages of success of their medial or lateral counterparts (Fig. 13.8) [11].

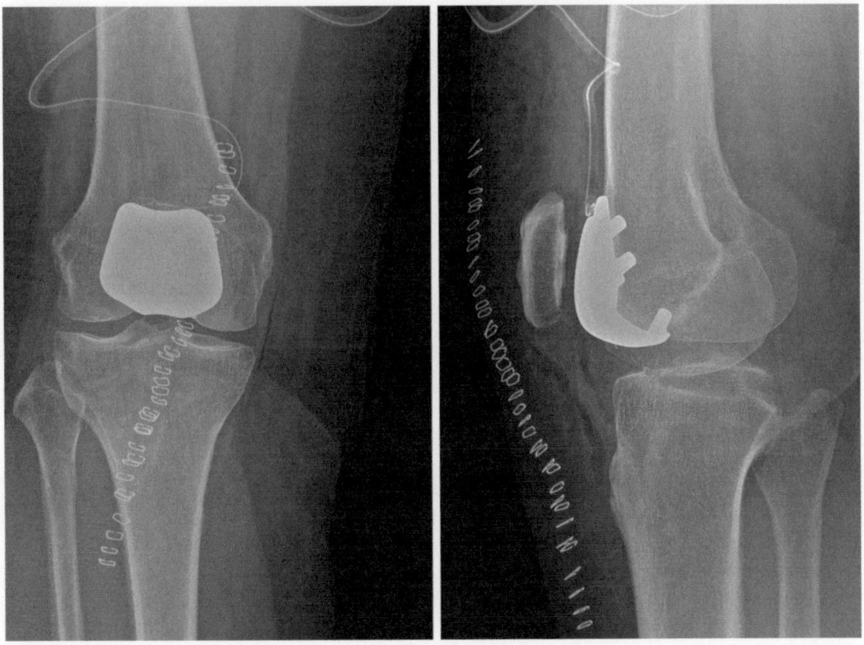

Fig. 13.8 Patellofemoral unicompartmental knee replacement

From a planning point of view, it must be pointed out that the implant choice reflects different positioning strategies. For onlay implants, the positioning should be flush with the native trochlea, with rotation determined by the native anatomy, while for inlay implants that replace the entire trochlea, they should be placed perpendicular to the AP axis and extends further proximal than the native trochlea.

In either case, external rotation of the patellofemoral component is unsuggested as it will decrease the patellar jump height, increasing the risk of lateral subluxation.

Take Home Messages

1. A complete radiographic examination of the knee is crucial in planning a unicompartmental knee replacement: long-standing AP and lateral X-ray of the knee are mandatory. Posterior tibial slope is one of the most important parameters to be evaluated.
2. In medial UKA the tibial cut is crucial. The most important indications are: (1) avoid overcorrection and (2) cut the minimal depth possible in order to restore the pre-osteoarthritic alignment.
3. The improper positioning of the femoral component in medial UKA is a frequent cause of early wear and loosening. Ideally, the points of contact between the polyethylene and the femoral component should lay on the rotational center of the component itself.

4. Lateral UKA accounts for 10% of UKA performed. In this procedure the positioning and sizing of the femoral component might be more difficult than in medial UKA. The femoral component should be never oversized and positioned as lateral as possible on the femoral condyle, without removing lateral osteophytes. As per the medial side, never overcorrect.

References

1. Crawford DA, Berend KR, Thienpont E. Unicompartmental knee arthroplasty: US and global perspectives. Orthop Clin North Am. 2020;51:147–59.
2. Zuiderbaan HA, van der List JP, Kleeblad LJ, Appelboom P, Kort NP, Pearle AD, Rademakers MV. Modern indications, results, and global trends in the use of unicompartmental knee arthroplasty and high tibial osteotomy in the treatment of isolated medial compartment osteoarthritis. Am J Orthop Belle Mead NJ. 2016;45:E355–61.
3. Aleto TJ, Berend ME, Ritter MA, Faris PM, Meneghini RM. Early failure of unicompartmental knee arthroplasty leading to revision. J Arthroplast. 2008;23:159–63.
4. Ahmad R, Patel A, Mandalia V, Toms A. Posterior tibial slope: effect on, and interaction with, knee kinematics. JBJS Rev. 2016;4:e31–6.
5. Chen Y, Ding J, Dai S, Yang J, Wang M, Tian T, Deng X, Li B, Cheng G, Liu J. Radiographic measurement of the posterior tibial slope in normal Chinese adults: a retrospective cohort study. BMC Musculoskelet Disord. 2022;23:386.
6. Vyas S, van Eck CF, Vyas N, Fu FH, Otsuka NY. Increased medial tibial slope in teenage pediatric population with open physes and anterior cruciate ligament injuries. Knee Surg Sports Traumatol Arthrosc. 2011;19:372–7.
7. Richardson AB, Morris MJ. Medial unicompartmental knee arthroplasty. Instr Course Lect. 2017;66:201–9.
8. Lo Presti M, Raspugli GF, Reale D, Iacono F, Zaffagnini S, Filardo G, Marcacci M. Early failure in medial unicondylar arthroplasty: radiographic analysis on the importance of joint line restoration. J Knee Surg. 2019;32:860–5.
9. Fratini S, Meena A, Alesi D, Cammisa E, Zaffagnini S, Marcheggiani Muccioli GM. Does implant design influence failure rate of lateral unicompartmental knee arthroplasty? A meta-analysis. J Arthroplast. 2022;37:985–992.e3.
10. Ollivier M, Abdel MP, Parratte S, Argenson J-N. Lateral unicondylar knee arthroplasty (UKA): contemporary indications, surgical technique, and results. Int Orthop. 2014;38:449–55.
11. Lustig S. Patellofemoral arthroplasty. Orthop Traumatol Surg Res OTSR. 2014;100:S35–43.

Preoperative Planning for Primary Total Knee Arthroplasty (Mechanical, Anatomic, and Kinematic Alignment)

14

D. Alesi, B. Al-Zubi, S. Fratini, E. Cammisa, M. La Verde, and Giulio Maria Marcheggiani Muccioli

14.1 Introduction

Proper knee alignment and soft tissue envelope integrity have been considered to be influential factors in determining the long-term outcomes and implant survival after total knee arthroplasty (TKA) [1]. Nowadays, several alignment options have been introduced in knee arthroplasty. Among them, the reference ones are mechanical alignment, anatomical alignment, and kinematic alignment [2]. In addition, the concept of hybrid alignment was recently introduced with the aim of optimizing the advantages of different types of alignment [2, 3]. Regardless of the choice of alignment, every patient requires a careful clinical and radiological assessment before knee replacement surgery; this preliminary study allows us to investigate the different characteristics and deformities presented by each patient and to be prepared for intra-operative challenges [4].

The preoperative clinical evaluation aims to analyze and quantify several parameters such as ligamentous laxity, flexion contracture, deformity reducibility, and preoperative range of motion (ROM).

The evaluation of the ligamentous laxity guides the surgeon in the choice of appropriate implant constraint [5]. For example, a valid posterior cruciate ligament will allow the implant of a cruciate retaining arthroplasty. Large varus or valgus deformities can lead to collateral ligamentous contractures on the concave side and laxity on the convex side; therefore, performing a varus–valgus stress test at 0° and 30° of knee flexion can guide the choice of implant constraint [6–8]. Flexion contractures ranging from 5° up to 20–30° can occur in case of severe osteoarthritis; these cases require precautions to be taken into account before surgery: to achieve

D. Alesi · B. Al-Zubi · S. Fratini · E. Cammisa · M. La Verde
G. M. Marcheggiani Muccioli (✉)
2nd Orthopedic and Traumatologic Clinic, IRCCS Istituto Ortopedico Rizzoli, Bologna, Italy
e-mail: giulio.marcheggiani2@unibo.it

G. M. Marcheggiani Muccioli et al. (eds.), *Easy Planning in Elective Primary Orthopedic Procedures*, https://doi.org/10.1007/978-3-031-77006-7_14

full extension it will be necessary to plan for a larger distal femur cut. Deformity reducibility predicts the need to perform ligament release in order to obtain balanced gaps [9]. No less important is the assessment of preoperative ROM; the literature shows how this correlates with postoperative ROM [10]. Therefore, the patient should be warned about the difficulty of obtaining a full ROM in case of limited preoperative ROM. This limitation is, in fact, partly due to inveterate contracture of the extensor apparatus and joint capsule, which can only be partially corrected during surgery.

14.2 Radiographic Examination

Radiographic examination is essential before any total knee arthroplasty (TKA) to assess the axis of the lower limbs and the grade of osteoarthritis of each knee; these radiological studies include a long-standing view of the knee for overall coronal alignment, lateral knee radiographs, and skyline radiographs (Merchant view) [4, 11]. A long-standing view of the knee allows to draw the femoral and tibial anatomical and mechanical axes, the difference between them, namely the anatomical mechanical angle (AMA), the hip-knee-ankle (HKA) angle, and the Paley's angles (mechanical medial proximal tibial angle—mMPTA, mechanical lateral distal femoral angle—mLDFA, joint line convergence angle—JLCA), which allow detailed analysis of the cause of the deformity (Fig. 14.1) [12]. Furthermore, a long-standing view of the knee allows us to assess the presence of femoral or tibial extra-articular deformities, the correctability of which at the intra-articular level is influenced by their size and proximity to the joint. The closer the deformity is to the joint, the more its correction may alter the joint line or be proximal to the epicondyles [13].

Lateral knee radiographs allow us to analyze the tibial slope, patellar height, anterior and posterior femoral offset and to evaluate the presence of posterior osteophytes (Fig. 14.2). Regarding the tibial slope, there is no consensus regarding the calculation method. The best compromise is obtained by subtracting the angle between the tangent to the tibial medial condyle and the long axis of the tibia to 90°. The long axis of the tibia is determined by drawing a line passing through the center of two circles: one midway between the anterior and posterior border of the tibia at the level of the tibial tubercle and the other 5 cm distal to the tubercle [14].

Lastly, the skyline radiographs show the patellofemoral joint, allowing measurement of the patellar tilt angle, sulcus angle, and patellar shift (Fig. 14.3).

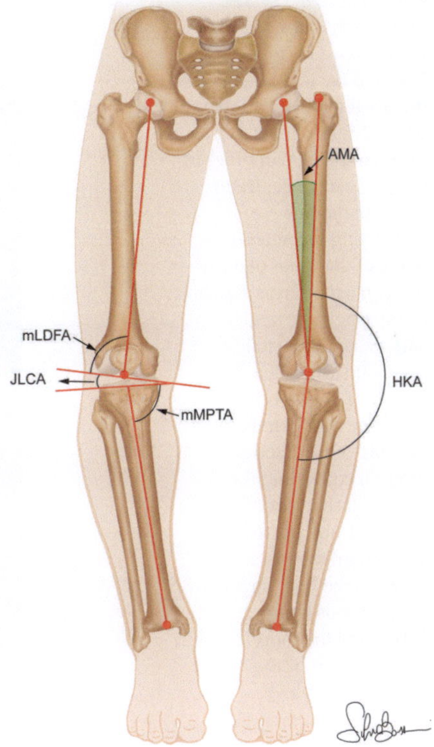

Fig. 14.1 Angles around the knee. On the right leg, femoral and tibial mechanical axes (red axes), joint line convergence angle (JLCA), mechanical medial proximal tibial angle (mMPTA), and mechanical lateral distal femoral angle (mLDFA) are reported. On the left leg, the anatomical mechanical angle (AMA), or the angle between the anatomical and mechanical femoral axis, and the hip knee ankle (HKA), or the angle between mechanical femoral and tibial axes are reported. Copyright of Silvia Bassini, 2024. All rights reserved

14.3 Alignment

14.3.1 Mechanical Alignment

Since the introduction of TKA in the 1970s, mechanical alignment (MA) has remained the most adopted alignment technique for TKA, popularized by Insall and Scott [1].

The primary goals of MA are to obtain a stable knee with a neutral lower limb alignment fundamental for successful clinical outcomes and implant survivorship [10]. The joint line is oriented perpendicular to the neutral mechanical axis of the limb and the femoral component is expected to be frontally and axially aligned with the trans-epicondylar axis (TEA), which then becomes the flexion–extension axis of the knee. The aim is not to restore the constitutional knee anatomy but rather to obtain a "biomechanically friendly prosthetic knee," which aims at reducing the adduction moment and distributing the load more evenly on the tibial compartments to prevent instability, accelerated polyethylene wear, and early implant loosening [15].

Before the surgery, AMA must be calculated on long-standing radiographs of the knee; this makes it possible to assess the resection angle to be set for the distal

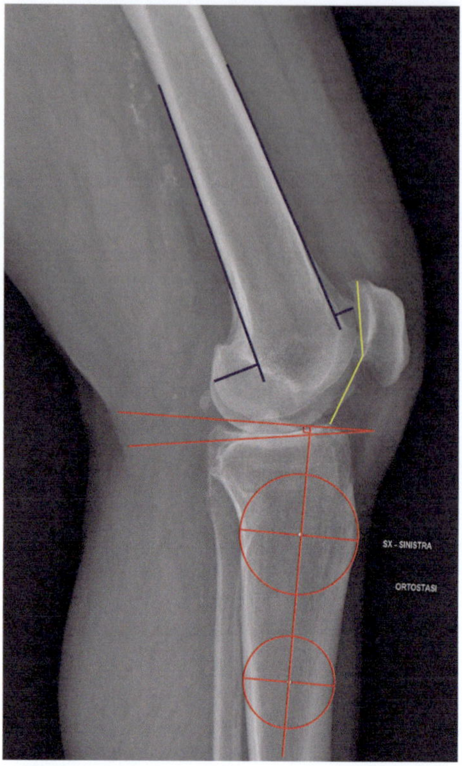

Fig. 14.2 Lateral knee radiographs showing the tibial slope (the angle between the line tangent to the tibial plateau and the tibial longitudinal axis), patellar height according to Caton Deschamps (ratio between the line connecting the anterior angle of the tibial plateau to the most inferior aspect of the patellar articular surface and the patellar articular surface length), anterior femoral offset (distance between the line tangent to the anterior femoral cortex and the more anterior part of the trochlea), and posterior femoral offset (distance between the line tangent to the posterior femoral cortex and the more posterior part of the femoral condyles)

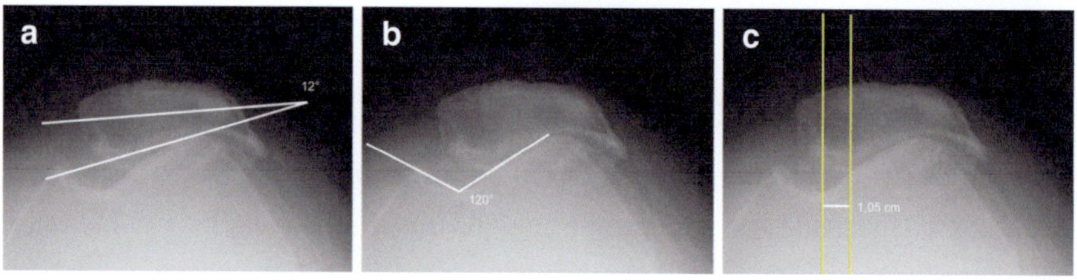

Fig. 14.3 Skyline radiographs showing the patellofemoral joint, allowing measurement of the patellar tilt angle (**a**), sulcus angle (**b**), and patellar shift (**c**)

femoral cut (using an angle equal to AMA will provide a neutral mechanical aligned TKA). This angle is usually set between 5° and 7°. In the presence of a severe knee deformity, a 1–2° under correction of the deformity could help in ligament balancing without rising up the risk of deformity recurrence (Fig. 14.4a) [3].

It is possible to calculate the thickness of the distal femoral cut by drawing the mechanical axis of the femur and tracing a perpendicular line. The minimum resection thickness for the distal femoral cut is usually considered 9 mm (from the medial condyle in a varus knee and from the lateral condyle in a valgus one (Fig. 14.4b)). However, it depends on the prosthetic model used and must be increased in the case

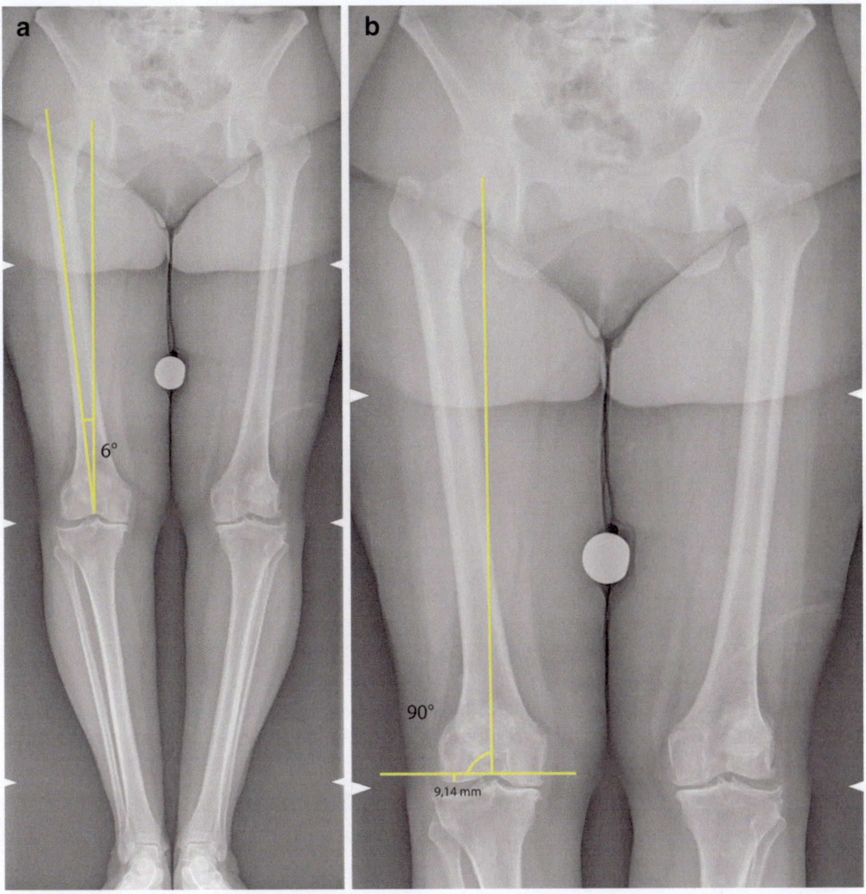

Fig. 14.4 (**a**) Anatomical mechanical angle used to calculate the resection angle to be set for the distal femoral cut. (**b**) Distal femoral cut thickness calculated positioning a line perpendicular to femoral mechanical axis minimum 9 mm proximally from the distal aspect of the unaffected condyle

of flexion contracture. It must be kept in mind, however, that increasing the thickness of the distal femoral cut can generate patella baja, which is among the factors leading to mid-flexion instability as it unbalances the extension gap with respect to the flexion gap.

Drawing the mechanical axis of the tibia and tracing a perpendicular line, it is possible to calculate the thickness of the tibial cut, it would be 9–10 mm on the healthy or 2 mm on the worn compartment (Fig. 14.5).

Traditionally, neutral mechanical alignment is undertaken to achieve postoperative limb alignment to within 3° of neutral to the mechanical axis. Measured resections or gap balancing techniques are used to equalize flexion–extension gaps and achieve equipoise in mediolateral soft-tissue tension [1]. Another important parameter is the joint line convergence angle (JLCA), which is measured to evaluate knee

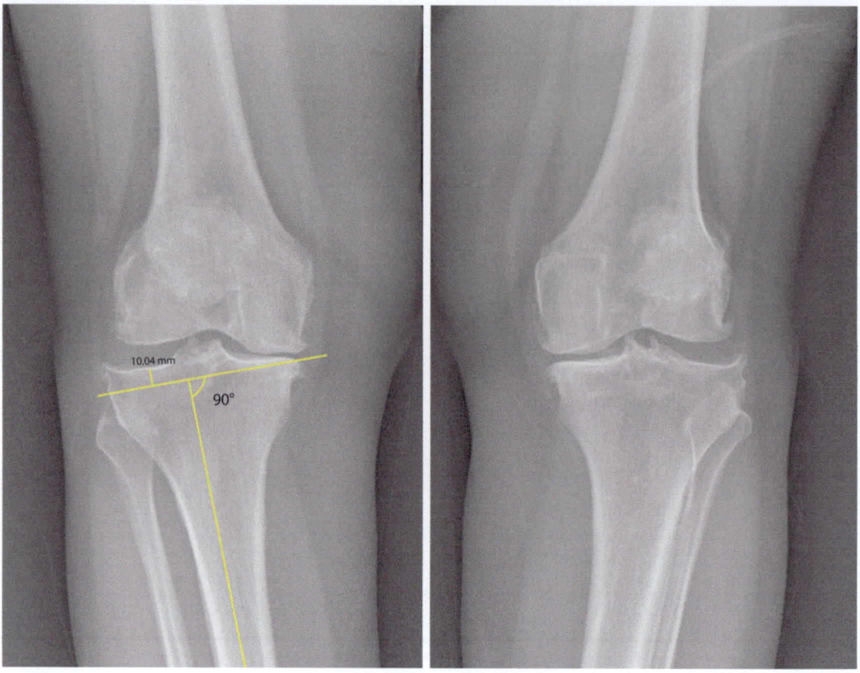

Fig. 14.5 Proximal tibial cut thickness calculated positioning a line perpendicular to the tibial mechanical axis 9–10 mm distally from the healthy or 2 mm distally from the worn compartment

joint congruity, as the angle formed between a line tangential to the distal femoral condyles and the tibial plateau; an excessive inclination (>5°) likely will require ligament release (Fig. 14.6).

Lateral knee radiographs show preoperative posterior tibial slope (PTS), which must be set according to the design used. It is usually set to 5° in the case of cruciate-retaining prostheses (to increase flexion) and 3° to 0° in the case of posterior-stabilized implants. The posterior and anterior offsets provide information on the choice of size. It must be kept in mind that in the case of posterior reference implants, the posterior resection will be constant, while the thickness of the anterior cut will increase as the size decreases. The opposite applies in the case of anterior reference implants (more common nowadays).

It must be kept in mind that excessive anterior compartment bulk can create an overstuff on the patella, which can cause pain. Furthermore, anteriorizing the femoral component opens the flexion gap and it is one of the causes that can lead to mid-flexion instability, as well as anterior pain.

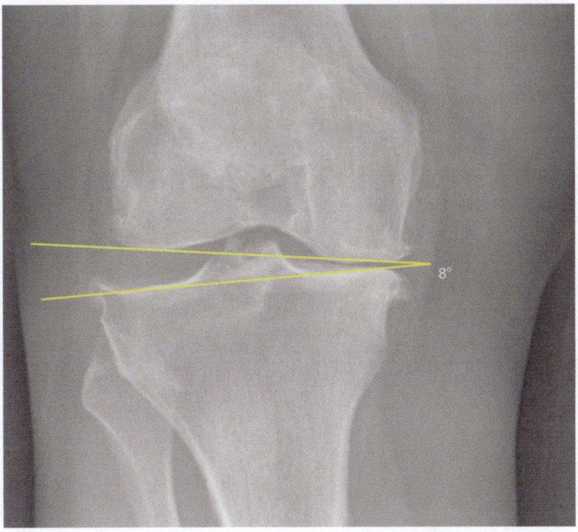

Fig. 14.6 Joint line convergence angle (JLCA) measured to evaluate knee joint congruity, as the angle formed between a line tangential to the distal femoral condyles and the tibial plateau; an excessive inclination (>5°) likely will require ligament release

14.3.2 Anatomic Alignment

Described and popularized by Hungerford and Krackow in the 1980s, anatomic alignment aims to maintain the anatomical limb alignment so that the joint line is parallel to the ground when standing [2]. A 3° varus tibial cut and a 3° valgus femoral cut allow to recreate a 6° valgus joint line (Fig. 14.7).

However, due to the high incidence of outliers in the coronal implant positioning, which has been seen to correlate with early failure, this alignment technique has been progressively abandoned, with the introduction of implants with an anatomic joint line but which can be implanted with mechanical alignment (anatomic-alignment-like technique) or the increasingly popular kinematic alignment.

14.3.3 Kinematic Alignment (and Restricted Kinematic Alignment)

Kinematic alignment (KA) was introduced in 2006 by Howell and the engineer Hull, with the aim to preserve the constitutional alignment of the knee and to promote physiological kinematics [16]. KA should allow patients to achieve better function and less pain after TKA, reducing the incidence of mid-flexion instability and stiffness, and improving knee kinematics [17]. Mechanical and anatomical alignments keep the implants in a "neutral" position by changing the patient's original alignment, in some cases creating instability or tension on ligament structures that cannot be modified, which obviously affects the result and patient satisfaction [17]. Kinematic alignment has been defined as "joint line surgery" in which the bone cuts aim to resurface the worn joint surfaces, preserving the native anatomy of the knee; this results in the alignment of the components to the kinematic axes of the

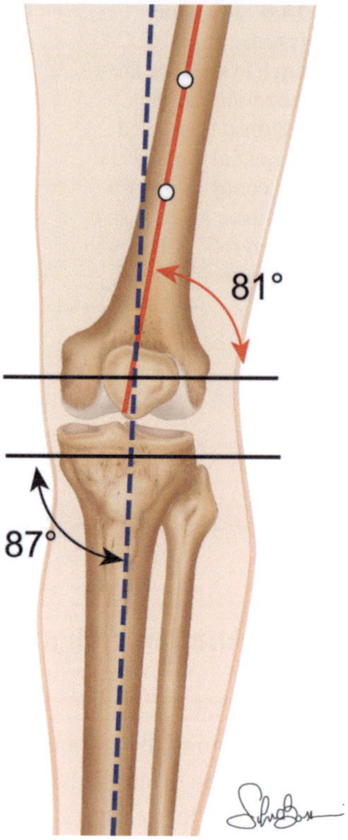

Fig. 14.7 Bone cuts in anatomic alignment. A 3° varus tibial cut (87° mMPTA) and 9° valgus femoral cut with respect to the femoral anatomical axis (81° anatomical lateral distal femoral angle (aLDFA)) allow to recreate a 6° valgus joint line. Copyright of Silvia Bassini, 2024. All rights reserved

knee and maintains the soft tissue envelope, and minimizes the need for ligament release. The implant must replace the pre-arthritic thickness of bone and cartilage with an equivalent metal thickness [18]. The components are aligned on the three knee axes that dictate its kinematics: the femoral flexion axis (cylindrical or transcondylar axis), the tibial rotation axis (longitudinal axis), and the patellar flexion axis (Fig. 14.8).

The femoral component is aligned parallel to the femoral cylindrical axis in the frontal and axial planes and follows the distal femur's physiological curvature in the sagittal plane. The tibial component is aligned parallel to the femoral cylindrical axis in the frontal plane, the medial tibial plateau in the sagittal plane, and the anteroposterior tibial axis in the axial plane.

The thickness of the bone cuts must be equal to that of the prosthetic component that will be implanted. In this calculation, cartilage wear, which is defined as 2 mm at the level of the distal femur and 1 mm at the level of the posterior–lateral condyle in the valgus knee, and saw thickness, which is approximated to 1 mm, must be considered. For example, considering a varus knee, the resection of the medial femoral condyle will be 6 mm + 2 mm of cartilage wear +1 mm of saw = 9 mm. In contrast, the thickness of the lateral condyle, where there is no wear, will be 8 mm + 1 mm saw = 9 mm, and so on. This concept is known as "calipered

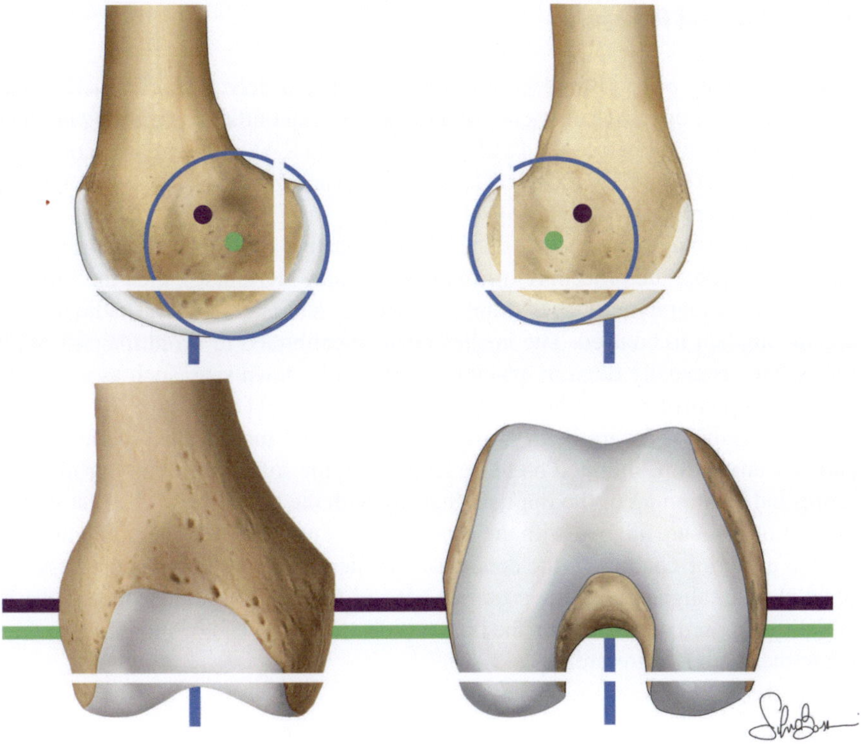

Fig. 14.8 Axes used in kinematic alignment. The femoral flexion axis (green line on frontal and axial plane and green dot on lateral plane), the tibial rotation axis (blue line on frontal and axial plane), and the patellar flexion axis (purple line on frontal and axial plane and purple dot on lateral plane).

resection" because bone cuts must be measured, and it is one of the cornerstone concepts of KA [19].

In patients with extreme knee/lower limb constitutional anatomy, it is possible to retain a KA philosophy while adjusting the alignment of the components to reduce and make the residual deformity acceptable. This hybrid alignment technique is gaining considerable interest and is known as "restricted KA" (rKA) [20]. This technique can be applied when the patient has considerable constitutional lower limb deformity; rKA provides to correct the tibial cut to no more than 5° from the mechanical axis and to apply the concept of KA on the femoral side. The resulting HKA must not deviate more than 3° from the neutral alignment to reduce the risks of implant failure [16].

14.4 Digital Planning

Digital planning prior to total knee arthroplasty is a widely adopted practice that aims to improve operative efficiency and reduce clinical outliers. Predicting implant size and positioning before total knee arthroplasty (TKA), although less common, could increase operating room efficiency by reducing the necessary equipment needed for the procedure [21].

Digital planning is commonly done using dedicated software. The first step is to select the appropriate procedure (primary or revision TKA, side), then the surgeon selects the radiographic images (long leg standing and lateral–lateral radiographs) and the implant to be used. The images must be calibrated to avoid magnification errors. This is usually done by placing a marker of known size, such as a 32 mm head of a hip prosthesis, within the X-ray field (Fig. 14.9) [11, 22].

The planning software helps the surgeon mark and measure key points in the patient's anatomy. Calibrated on those landmarks, the software initially proposes a sizing and positioning of the implant. Starting with the lateral view, the first step is to position a square aligned with the anterior cortex of the femur, including the distal and posterior contour of the condyles. Another square is positioned across the tibial plateau, aligned with the posterior edge of the tibia. A default tibial slope is initially proposed depending on the implant selected, but it can be modified according to the surgeon's preferences.

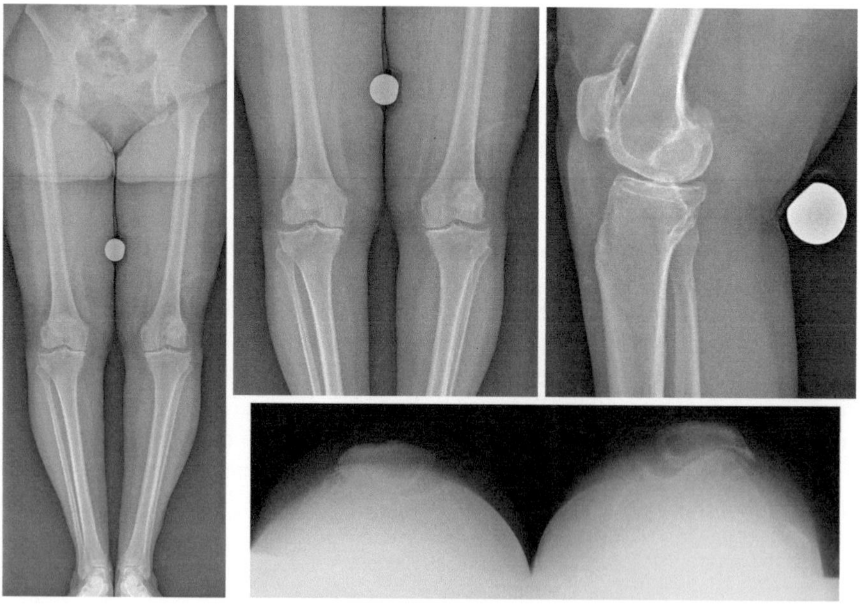

Fig. 14.9 Radiological series used for digital planning. The images are calibrated placing a marker of known size, such as a 32 mm head of a hip prosthesis, within the X-ray field

On the AP view, a box is positioned with the corners contouring the edges of the medial and lateral cortex to identify the anatomical axis of the femur. At this point, a line is positioned tangent to the distal femoral condyles. The angle between this line and the femoral anatomical axis can be adjusted as the surgeon prefers. This will determine the varus–valgus orientation of the distal femoral cut.

On the tibial side, the same process as the femoral side is performed to identify the tibial anatomical axis. Furthermore, the medial and lateral borders of the tibial plateau are identified. At this point, medial and lateral femoral and tibial cut depth is selected (Fig. 14.10).

The next step is the templating, where the software, calibrated on the measurements performed in the planning step, proposes an initial sizing and the positioning of the implant on AP and LL view (Fig. 14.11). Anyway, the surgeon is free to move from one size to another or to modify the implant positioning according to its preferences. The software will warn of possible matching incompatibilities.

Once the surgeon is satisfied with the templating, it can be saved and printed.

Nowadays, although with extended time, surgeons are trying to pass from two-dimensional (2D) planning accuracy with digital radiographs to a novel imaging technology that generates a three-dimensional (3D) model from 2D radiographs and CT scans [23]. Proper coronal alignment of TKA components is generally accepted to be an important factor in long-term implant survival; the 2D planning method used the distal femoral valgus angle of resection based on the hip–knee–ankle (HKA) radiograph combined, for example, with neutral tibial resection angle to achieve a neutral mechanical axis. 3D templating proved to have very high accuracy for the actual implant size prediction. Compared to this, as shown in different studies, 2D digital planning is an accurate method to approximately (±1 size) determine the size of TKA components but can only predict the actual implant in about 50% of the cases, while 3D planning is accurate in predicting the correct implant size in

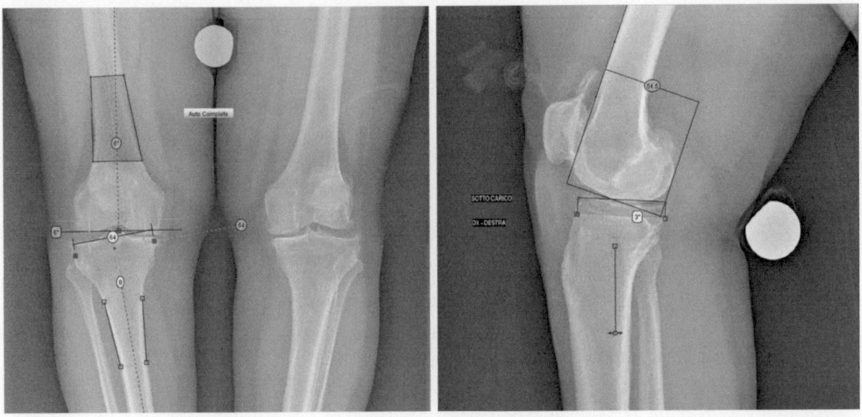

Fig. 14.10 Anteroposterior and laterolateral digital planning. A series of measurements are performed to identify anatomical and mechanical axes of femur and tibia, thickness and orientation of resections, anteroposterior femoral and tibial depth, and tibial slope

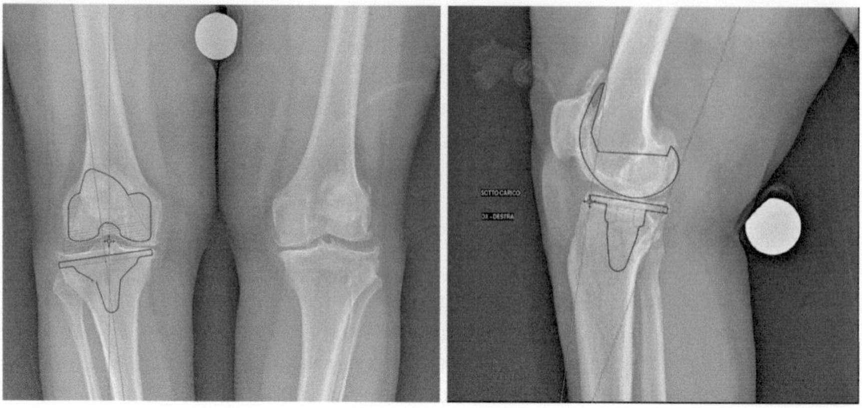

Fig. 14.11 Templating proposed after completion of digital planning. The surgeon is free to modify the implant orientation and to move from one size to another. The software will warn of possible matching incompatibilities

100% of the cases. Therefore, 3D planning appears to be the future and, in some cases, even the present of preoperative analysis that every patient should have before undergoing a TKA [24, 25].

Take Home Messages

1. The preoperative radiographic evaluation of a TKA must include a long-standing view of the knee for overall coronal alignment, lateral knee radiographs, and skyline radiographs (Merchant view).
2. Mechanical, anatomical, and kinematic alignment are all valuable options for TKA positioning and planning.
3. Mechanical alignment is still the gold standard, a good experience with this approach is desirable before moving to anatomical and kinematic ones.
4. Calibrated measurement of the bone cuts is desirable to understand if there is a true matching between the planning and the surgery.

References

1. Scuderi GR, Scott WN, Tchejeyan GH. The Insall legacy in total knee arthroplasty. Clin Orthop. 2001;392:3–14. https://doi.org/10.1097/00003086-200111000-00002.
2. Rivière C, Iranpour F, Auvinet E, et al. Alignment options for total knee arthroplasty: a systematic review. Orthop Traumatol Surg Res OTSR. 2017;103(7):1047–56. https://doi.org/10.1016/j.otsr.2017.07.010.
3. Begum FA, Kayani B, Magan AA, Chang JS, Haddad FS. Current concepts in total knee arthroplasty: mechanical, kinematic, anatomical, and functional alignment. Bone Jt Open. 2021;2(6):397–404. https://doi.org/10.1302/2633-1462.26.BJO-2020-0162.R1.

4. Haas H, Weber CD. Preoperative evaluation of patients undergoing Total joint arthroplasty – what is essential? Z Orthopadie Unfallchirurgie. 2017;155(5):549–55. https://doi.org/10.1055/s-0043-114418.
5. Ishii Y, Noguchi H, Sato J, et al. Alignment evaluation using different distal reference points after total knee arthroplasty. J Orthop. 2021;25:186–90. https://doi.org/10.1016/j.jor.2021.05.013.
6. Rossi R, Rosso F, Cottino U, Dettoni F, Bonasia DE, Bruzzone M. Total knee arthroplasty in the valgus knee. Int Orthop. 2014;38(2):273–83. https://doi.org/10.1007/s00264-013-2227-4.
7. Alesi D, Meena A, Fratini S, et al. Total knee arthroplasty in valgus knee deformity: is it still a challenge in 2021? Musculoskelet Surg. Published online February,. 2021;15:1. https://doi.org/10.1007/s12306-021-00695-x.
8. Rossi R, Cottino U, Bruzzone M, Dettoni F, Bonasia DE, Rosso F. Total knee arthroplasty in the varus knee: tips and tricks. Int Orthop. 2019;43(1):151–8. https://doi.org/10.1007/s00264-018-4116-3.
9. Jaffe WL, Dundon JM, Camus T. Alignment and balance methods in total knee arthroplasty. J Am Acad Orthop Surg. 2018;26(20):709–16. https://doi.org/10.5435/JAAOS-D-16-00428.
10. Parratte S, Pagnano MW, Trousdale RT, Berry DJ. Effect of postoperative mechanical axis alignment on the fifteen-year survival of modern, cemented total knee replacements. J Bone Joint Surg Am. 2010;92(12):2143–9. https://doi.org/10.2106/JBJS.I.01398.
11. Tanzer M, Makhdom AM. Preoperative planning in primary total knee arthroplasty. J Am Acad Orthop Surg. 2016;24(4):220–30. https://doi.org/10.5435/JAAOS-D-14-00332.
12. Antony J, Tetsworth K, Hohmann E. Influence of sagittal plane component alignment on kinematics after total knee arthroplasty. Knee Surg Sports Traumatol Arthrosc. 2017;25(6):1686–91. https://doi.org/10.1007/s00167-016-4098-x.
13. Steer R, Tippett B, Khan RN, Collopy D, Clark G. A prospective randomised control trial comparing functional with mechanical axis alignment in total knee arthroplasty: study protocol for an investigator initiated trial. Trials. 2021;22(1):523. https://doi.org/10.1186/s13063-021-05433-z.
14. Vyas S, van Eck CF, Vyas N, Fu FH, Otsuka NY. Increased medial tibial slope in teenage pediatric population with open physes and anterior cruciate ligament injuries. Knee Surg Sports Traumatol Arthrosc. 2011;19(3):372–7. https://doi.org/10.1007/s00167-010-1216-z.
15. Takashima Y, Matsumoto T, Takayama K, et al. Comparison of clinical and biomechanical outcomes between the kinematic and mechanical alignment methods in total knee arthroplasty: protocol for a multicenter randomized controlled trial. Contemp Clin Trials Commun. 2021;22:100775. https://doi.org/10.1016/j.conctc.2021.100775.
16. Weber P, Gollwitzer H. Kinematic alignment in total knee arthroplasty. Oper Orthop Traumatol. 2021;33(6):525–37. https://doi.org/10.1007/s00064-021-00729-4.
17. Sappey-Marinier E, Pauvert A, Batailler C, et al. Kinematic versus mechanical alignment for primary total knee arthroplasty with minimum 2 years follow-up: a systematic review. SICOT-J. 2020;6:18. https://doi.org/10.1051/sicotj/2020014.
18. Liu B, Feng C, Tu C. Kinematic alignment versus mechanical alignment in primary total knee arthroplasty: an updated meta-analysis of randomized controlled trials. J Orthop Surg. 2022;17(1):201. https://doi.org/10.1186/s13018-022-03097-2.
19. Rivière C, Villet L, Jeremic D, Vendittoli PA. What you need to know about kinematic alignment for total knee arthroplasty. Orthop Traumatol Surg Res OTSR. 2021;107(1S):102773. https://doi.org/10.1016/j.otsr.2020.102773.
20. Risitano S, Cacciola G, Sabatini L, et al. Restricted kinematic alignment in primary total knee arthroplasty: a systematic review of radiographic and clinical data. J Orthop. 2022;33:37–43. https://doi.org/10.1016/j.jor.2022.06.014.
21. Del Gaizo D, Soileau ES, Lachiewicz PF. Value of preoperative templating for primary total knee arthroplasty. J Knee Surg. 2009;22(4):284–93. https://doi.org/10.1055/s-0030-1247765.
22. Khalifa AA, Mullaji AB, Mostafa AM, Farouk OA. A protocol to systematic radiographic assessment of primary total knee arthroplasty. Orthop Res Rev. 2021;13:95–106. https://doi.org/10.2147/ORR.S320372.

23. Ettinger M, Claassen L, Paes P, Calliess T. 2D versus 3D templating in total knee arthroplasty. Knee. 2016;23(1):149–51. https://doi.org/10.1016/j.knee.2015.08.014.
24. Klag EA, Lizzio VA, Charters MA, et al. Increased accuracy in templating for total knee arthroplasty using 3D models generated from radiographs. J Knee Surg. Published online March 3,. 2022;36:837. https://doi.org/10.1055/s-0042-1743496.
25. Gopurathingal AA, Bhonsle S. Inter-observer and intra-observer reliability of 2D radiograph-based valgus cut angle measurement in preoperative planning for primary total knee arthroplasty. Cureus. 2021;13(1):e12788. https://doi.org/10.7759/cureus.12788.

Preoperative Planning in Robotic-Assisted Knee Arthroplasty

15

Heather J. Roberts and Nicholas A. Bedard

15.1 Introduction

Robotic assistance in total and unicompartmental knee arthroplasty has been available in some form since the early 1990s [1]. Robotic-assistance improves precision in executing a preoperative plan [2–6], although this has not been shown to translate to improved long-term outcomes [7]. Robotic-assistance has been shown to improve early functional outcomes, facilitate early discharge, and decrease postoperative pain [8, 9]. In the Australian joint replacement registry, robotic-assisted total and unicompartmental knee arthroplasty are associated with lower rates of revision compared to traditional instrumentation [10]. However, robotic-assisted knee arthroplasty procedures are associated with longer operative times and increased cost, particularly for image-based systems that require preoperative three-dimensional imaging [11]. Despite this, robotic-assisted knee arthroplasty is increasing in popularity, with a steady annual increase in utilization [10, 12–14].

Preoperative planning for robotic-assisted knee arthroplasty follows largely the same guidelines as for knee arthroplasty performed with manual instrumentation. While the surgeon controls the preoperative plan in both situations, robotic assistance has the potential to improve precision in executing the plan. Robotics also allows for consideration of additional variables in generating the preoperative plan, such as the position of the native trochlea and native distal femoral dimensions in sizing and placing the femoral component. Robotic-assisted knee arthroplasty is compatible with various alignment goals, including mechanical alignment, kinematic alignment, or a variation of either.

In some robotic knee arthroplasty systems, preoperative planning for robotic-assisted total knee arthroplasty occurs both prior to incision and prior to making

H. J. Roberts · N. A. Bedard (✉)
Department of Orthopedic Surgery, Mayo Clinic, Rochester, MN, USA
e-mail: Bedard.Nicholas@mayo.edu

G. M. Marcheggiani Muccioli et al. (eds.), *Easy Planning in Elective Primary Orthopedic Procedures*, https://doi.org/10.1007/978-3-031-77006-7_15

bony cuts. In those systems, a preliminary bony cut plan is generated prior to incision based on preoperative imaging. The pre-incision plan can then be adjusted as needed after assessing intraoperative ligamentous laxity to finalize the surgical plan prior to bony resection. This intraoperative pre-resection planning occurs in both image-based and imageless robotic technologies.

15.2 Pre-Incision Planning: Image-Based Robotic Systems

Current image-based robotic systems rely on preoperative three-dimensional imaging, which is used in conjunction with standard anteroposterior (AP) and lateral radiographs to develop the surgical plan. While AP and lateral X-rays can be used to template sagittal and coronal alignment, planning with three-dimensional preoperative imaging allows for consideration of additional parameters, including the rotational position of the tibial and femoral components. For example, without advanced imaging, femoral component rotation can be determined intraoperatively using traditional anatomic landmarks such as the transepicondylar axis or posterior condylar axis. With three-dimensional imaging, the surgeon can additionally consider rotating the femoral component to match the native trochlea position to optimize patellofemoral kinematics while simultaneously considering the restoration of posterior femoral condylar offset. For the tibia, preoperative three-dimensional imaging can be used for sizing of the tibial tray to optimize tibial plateau coverage in addition to considering tibial component rotation relative to the native plateau and tibial tubercle.

Each surgeon may choose how to prioritize these anatomic parameters based on operative goals. For total knee arthroplasty, our preferred method of preoperative planning is to start with neutral mechanical axis alignment and neutral tibial resection (Fig. 15.1). We then assess femoral component rotation and anteroposterior positioning to restore posterior femoral condylar curvature and offset, particularly for the medial side (Fig. 15.2a), adjusting flexion of the femoral component as needed to avoid notching (Fig. 15.2b). We assess the femoral component trochlea position relative to the native trochlea, both with respect to rotation and anteroposterior translation, with the goal of optimizing patellofemoral tracking and avoiding overstuffing the patellofemoral joint (Fig. 15.3). We set the distal femoral resection to match the thickness of the distal aspect of the femoral component, particularly on the medial side. For the tibia, we set the tibial component rotation by matching it with the midline of the tibial plateau. We then determine the size of the tibial component by selecting the largest size that does not overhang the tibial cortex (Fig. 15.4). We set the tibial slope based on the type of implant we plan to use. We start with neutral coronal alignment and adjust intraoperatively as needed to achieve balance in the coronal plane.

For unicompartmental knee arthroplasty, we select the size of the tibial component that maximizes anteroposterior coverage. We then align the component with the medial tibial cortex and evaluate where this places the lateral border of the tibial component (Fig. 15.5). We downsize the tibial component if it extends laterally to

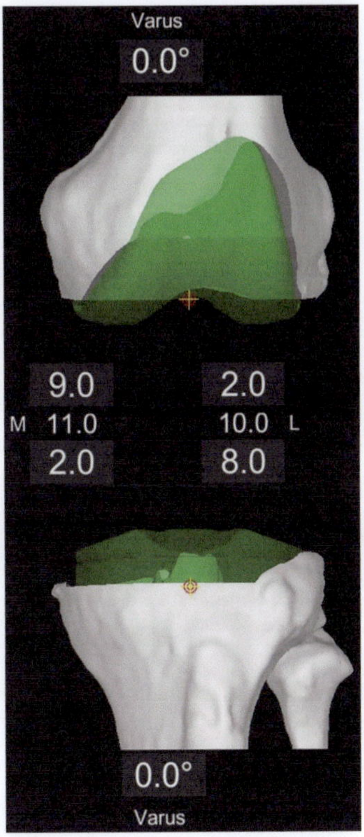

Fig. 15.1 Initial planning with neutral mechanical alignment of the femur and tibia

the peak of the medial tibial spine. Our preference is to cut the tibial component in 1° of varus for medial unicompartmental knee arthroplasties and 1° of valgus for lateral unicompartmental knee arthroplasties (Fig. 15.6). For the femoral component, we match the posterior condylar contour. We prefer the anterior flange of the femoral component to be 1–2 mm proud of the subchondral bone, accounting for up to 2 mm of cartilage in the intact trochlea (Fig. 15.7).

15.3 Intraoperative Registration and Pre-Resection Planning

For both image-based and imageless robotic-assisted knee arthroplasty, intraoperative registration is critical. Image-based robotic systems correlate to known three-dimensional anatomy, providing an additional check that imageless systems do not have. Therefore, precision in registration is particularly important in imageless robotic systems.

Both image-based and imageless systems fundamentally determine hip, knee, and ankle centers to aid in achieving the surgeon's alignment goals. Femoral and tibial bony landmarks are defined and stored relative to arrays fixed to the femur and tibia so that the robotic system can locate the knee in space, regardless of the

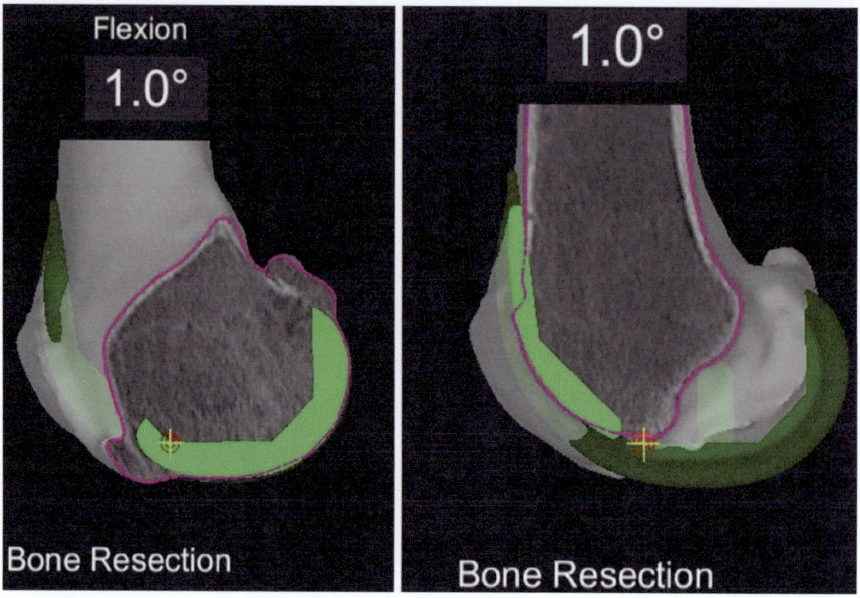

Fig. 15.2 Adjusting flexion of the femoral component helps match the posterior condyles (**a**) and avoid femoral notching (**b**)

Fig. 15.3 The femoral component is rotated so that the trochlea matches the native trochlea, optimizing patellofemoral kinematics

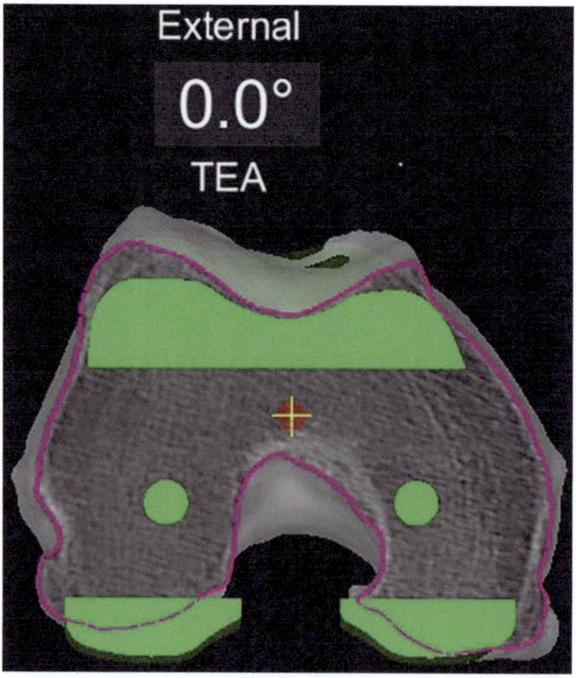

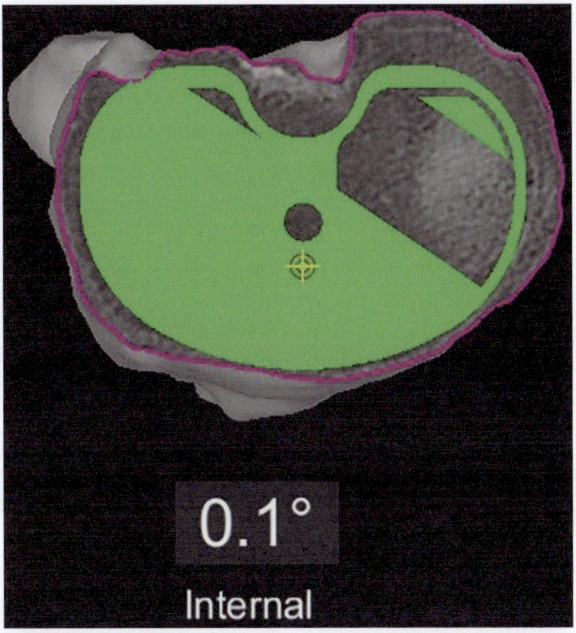

Fig. 15.4 The tibial component is selected to optimize size without overhang

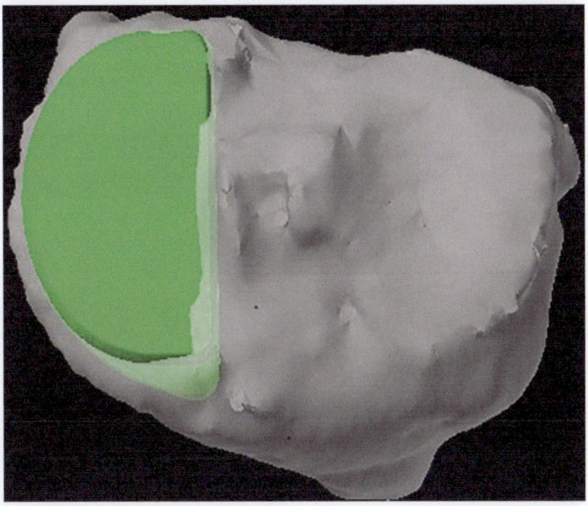

Fig. 15.5 The tibial component is sized to maximize anteroposterior coverage while staying medial to the peak of the medial tibial spine

position of the knee. Similar arrays are incorporated into the robotic arm to locate the position of the saw in space.

Once the knee is appropriately registered and prior to performing bony resections, the final stage of pre-resection planning is performed. It is important to assess the knee range of motion, including the presence of a flexion contracture, as well as coronal plane balance in extension and flexion. Steps that may affect balance, such as osteophyte removal and soft tissue releases, should be performed prior to

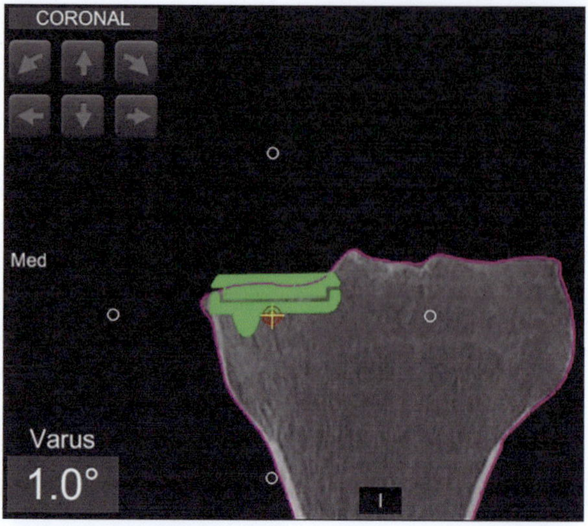

Fig. 15.6 Our preoperative plan includes 1° of varus on the tibial resection for a medial unicompartmental knee arthroplasty

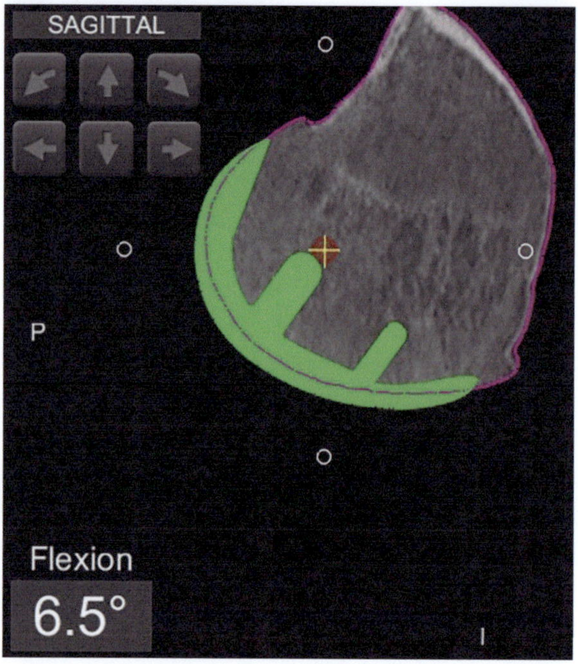

Fig. 15.7 Femoral sizing and position is adjusted to match the posterior condylar contour and position the anterior flange 1–2 mm proud of the subchondral bone

balancing. For example, if the release of the posterior cruciate ligament is planned with the implant being used, it should be released prior to pre-resection planning.

An advantage of robotic systems is that they provide a quantitative and precise assessment of medial and lateral gaps in extension and flexion, which can be used to adjust the planned bony resections to ensure a balanced knee at the completion of

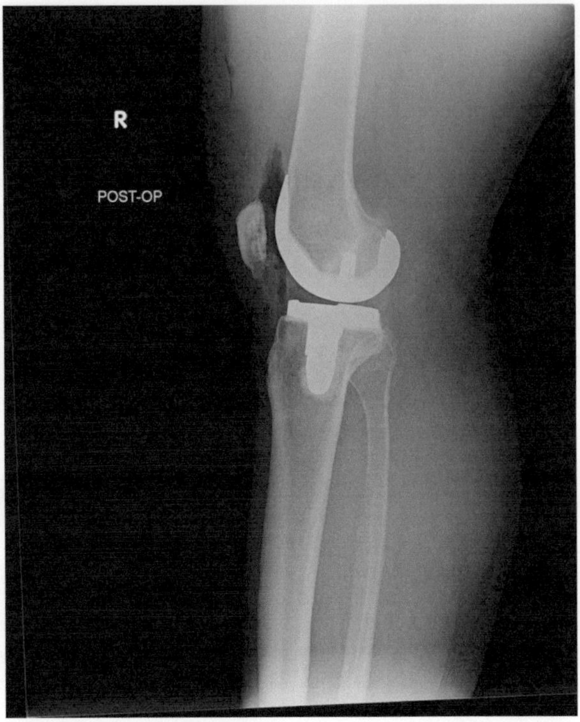

Fig. 15.8 Postoperative X-rays after robotic-assisted total knee arthroplasty

the case (Fig. 15.8). For image-based robotic systems, the initial pre-incision plan may be adjusted to account for these dynamic parameters observed intraoperatively. Similarly, with imageless robotic systems, bony resections and implant positions can be determined and adjusted at this step to optimize ultimate alignment and balancing. For example, the distal femoral resection may be increased to account for a flexion contracture; the femoral component can be flexed or extended to avoid notching; the femoral component can be rotated and/or the tibial slope can be adjusted to balance an imbalanced flexion gap; and both femoral and tibial components can be adjusted in the coronal plane to balance an imbalanced extension gap.

After performing bony resections, robotic systems can be used to evaluate whether ligamentous balancing goals have been achieved before implanting the final components. Should the balance of the knee be suboptimal, the intraoperative plan can be adjusted and bony resections repeated in order to achieve desired stability.

Take Home Messages

1. Robotic-assisted knee arthroplasty can allow for increased precision in executing a surgeon's desired alignment goals.

2. Robotic assistance provides information beyond standard preoperative X-ray templating because it provides the capacity to assess rotational alignment in addition to coronal and sagittal plane alignment.
3. Both image-based and imageless systems provide useful information to guide bony resections and optimize knee stability in total knee arthroplasty and unicompartmental knee arthroplasty.
4. Intraoperatively, robotic-assisted systems provide a quantitative assessment of the knee stability, allowing the surgeon to adjust bony resections and implant position as needed to optimize balance and carry out the surgeon's desired preoperative plan.

References

1. Jacofsky DJ, Allen M. Robotics in arthroplasty: a comprehensive review. J Arthroplast. 2016;31(10):2353–63. https://doi.org/10.1016/j.arth.2016.05.026.
2. Deckey DG, Rosenow CS, Verhey JT, et al. Robotic-assisted total knee arthroplasty improves accuracy and precision compared to conventional techniques. Bone Jt J. 2021;103-B(6 Supple A):74–80. https://doi.org/10.1302/0301-620X.103B6.BJJ-2020-2003.R1.
3. Hampp EL, Chughtai M, Scholl LY, et al. Robotic-arm assisted total knee arthroplasty demonstrated greater accuracy and precision to plan compared with manual techniques. J Knee Surg. 2019;32(3):239–50. https://doi.org/10.1055/s-0038-1641729.
4. Khlopas A, Sodhi N, Sultan AA, Chughtai M, Molloy RM, Mont MA. Robotic arm-assisted total knee arthroplasty. J Arthroplast. 2018;33(7):2002–6. https://doi.org/10.1016/j.arth.2018.01.060.
5. Negrín R, Duboy J, Iñiguez M, et al. Robotic-assisted vs conventional surgery in medial unicompartmental knee arthroplasty: a clinical and radiological study. Knee Surg Relat Res. 2021;33(1):5. https://doi.org/10.1186/s43019-021-00087-2.
6. Bell SW, Anthony I, Jones B, MacLean A, Rowe P, Blyth M. Improved accuracy of component positioning with robotic-assisted unicompartmental knee arthroplasty: data from a prospective, randomized controlled study. J Bone Jt Surg. 2016;98(8):627–35. https://doi.org/10.2106/JBJS.15.00664.
7. Kim YH, Yoon SH, Park JW. Does robotic-assisted TKA result in better outcome scores or long-term survivorship than conventional TKA? A randomized, Controlled Trial. Clin Orthop. 2020;478(2):266–75. https://doi.org/10.1097/CORR.0000000000000916.
8. Blyth MJG, Anthony I, Rowe P, Banger MS, MacLean A, Jones B. Robotic arm-assisted versus conventional unicompartmental knee arthroplasty: exploratory secondary analysis of a randomised controlled trial. Bone Jt Res. 2017;6(11):631–9. https://doi.org/10.1302/2046-3758.611.BJR-2017-0060.R1.
9. Kayani B, Konan S, Tahmassebi J, Pietrzak JRT, Haddad FS. Robotic-arm assisted total knee arthroplasty is associated with improved early functional recovery and reduced time to hospital discharge compared with conventional jig-based total knee arthroplasty: a prospective cohort study. Bone Jt J. 2018;100-B(7):930–7. https://doi.org/10.1302/0301-620X.100B7.BJJ-2017-1449.R1.
10. Australian Orthopaedic Association National Joint Replacement Registry 2022 Annual Report. AOANJRR. https://aoanjrr.sahmri.com/documents/10180/732916/AOA+2022+AR+Digital/f63ed890-36d0-c4b3-2e0b-7b63e2071b16. Accessed 17 Dec 2022.
11. Ponzio DY, Lonner JH. Preoperative mapping in unicompartmental knee arthroplasty using computed tomography scans is associated with radiation exposure and carries high cost. J Arthroplast. 2015;30(6):964–7. https://doi.org/10.1016/j.arth.2014.10.039.

12. Wang JC, Piple AS, Hill WJ, et al. Computer-navigated and robotic-assisted total knee arthroplasty: increasing in popularity without increasing complications. J Arthroplast. 2022;37(12):2358–64. https://doi.org/10.1016/j.arth.2022.06.014.
13. Bendich I, Kapadia M, Alpaugh K, Diane A, Vigdorchik J, Westrich G. Trends of utilization and 90-day complication rates for computer-assisted navigation and robotic assistance for total knee arthroplasty in the United States from 2010 to 2018. Arthroplasty Today. 2021;11:134–9. https://doi.org/10.1016/j.artd.2021.08.005.
14. Abdel MP, Meneghini RM, Berry DJ. Current practice trends in primary hip and knee arthroplasties among members of the American Association of Hip and Knee Surgeons: an update during the COVID-19 pandemic. J Arthroplast. 2021;36(7):S40–S44.e3. https://doi.org/10.1016/j.arth.2021.01.080.

Part VI

Osteotomy Around the Knee

A. Grassi

Patient Position and General Setting in Osteotomy Around the Knee

16

A. Grassi, E. Altovino, G. A. Lucidi, N. Maitan, M. Viotto, and Stefano Zaffagnini

16.1 Introduction

The knee osteotomy aims to correct malalignment of the mechanical axes of the lower extremities to correct, in most cases, varus or valgus deformities [1]. Alterations in the alignment of the limb result in an abnormal transmission of forces across intra- and extra-articular structures, predisposing to various joint pathologies [2]. Moreover, the load is shifted from the anatomic point of greatest pressure, which in a normal knee is the medial compartment for 60% of the weight-bearing [3].

The changing of the knee angles toward a varus or valgus type can wear down the cartilage of a compartment more and therefore speed up osteoarthritis [4].

To give a suitable surgical indication of knee osteotomies, it is essential to analyze as a first step the patient's medical history and perform the clinical examination; the patient should be inspected in an upright and supine position to examine the alignment of the lower limbs [5]. The second step is to analyze the X-rays of the knees, which must have been taken under weight-bearing with the leg in full extension in a long anteroposterior (AP) view [6].

There are different types of osteotomies: the correction of the malalignment can be performed by an osteotomy at the level of the femur or tibia, and it can be an opening wedge osteotomy or a closing wedge one, all depending on the level of the deformity and the surgeon's preferred technique [5].

A. Grassi (✉) · E. Altovino · G. A. Lucidi · N. Maitan · S. Zaffagnini
2nd Orthopedic and Traumatologic Clinic, IRCCS Istituto Ortopedico Rizzoli, Bologna, Italy
e-mail: alberto.grassi@ior.it

M. Viotto
IRCCS Istituto Ortopedico Rizzoli, S.C. Ortopedia Pediatria, Bologna, Italy

G. M. Marcheggiani Muccioli et al. (eds.), *Easy Planning in Elective Primary Orthopedic Procedures*, https://doi.org/10.1007/978-3-031-77006-7_16

16.2 Position and General Setting

Spinal or general anesthesia can be used for all osteotomies. After induction of anesthesia, to decrease the bleeding, a tourniquet should be applied to the thigh of the affected limb as far as possible from the surgical incision and inflated between 250 and 300 mmHg (Fig. 16.2) [7].

The patient is positioned in a supine way on a surgical table [8] (Fig. 16.1).

A sterile field is set up with appropriate disposable drapes in order to allow the evaluation of the lower limb axis and to allow free hip and knee motion during the surgery [9].

It is fundamental the presence of a radiology technician with an image intensifier in the operating room throughout the procedure for intraoperative fluoroscopy, usually placed on the opposite side of the surgeon [10].

As an aid throughout the surgery, the preoperative planning done previously can be printed or displayed on screens so that it can be compared during each step with the images shown by the image intensifier in real-time. The surgeon must consider that the planning X-rays were done with the patient standing and therefore under weight-bearing, while the images from the fluoroscope are done with the patient supine, so they do not consider ligamentous laxity.

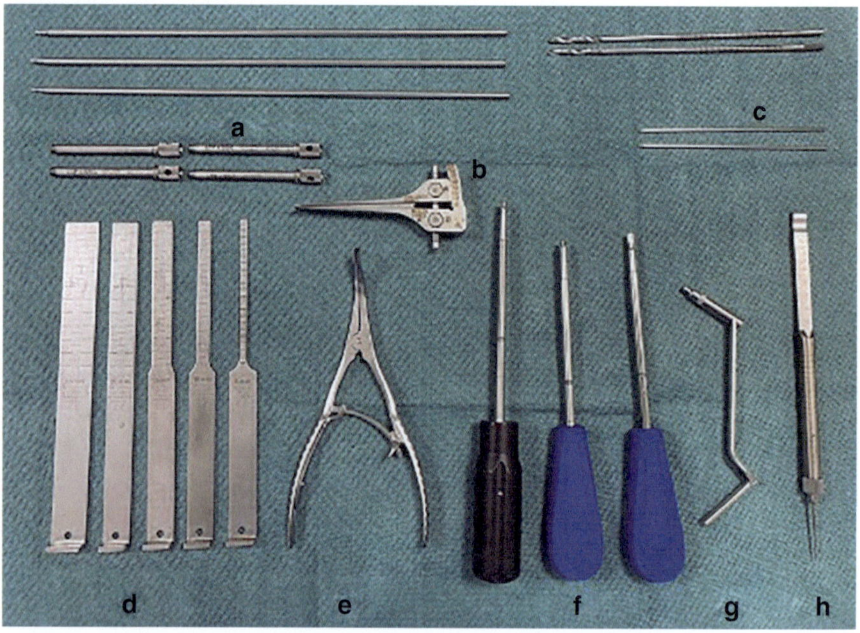

Fig. 16.2 Instruments needed for the osteotomies: (A) LCP guide sleeve, (B) spreader chisel, (C) K wires, (D) flat chisels (5–25 mm), (E) spreader, (F) screwdrivers, (G) soft tissue protector, (H) screw length meter

Positioning the patient in the proper way helps correct intraoperative imaging studies, therefore the contralateral limb should be lowered and the operative one may be raised on a foam bump [11].

During the first phase of the surgery, arthroscopy is often performed to evaluate the menisci and ligaments. Ancillary surgeries planned after careful preoperative clinical and radiological evaluation can be performed over this time of the surgery. For this reason, in addition to the instrumentation needed for open surgery, it is worth having all the tools required for case-specific-associated procedures in the operating room.

As previously mentioned, there are multiple techniques for an osteotomy around the knee to be executed, depending on where the deformity is located and the surgeon's preferred technique. The high tibial osteotomy (HTO) may be done medial or lateral to the tibia, and it could be either opening or closing wedge. To stabilize and decrease the implant and bone stress, systems with locking screws can be used [12].

The distal femur osteotomy (DFO) can be performed lateral or medial and it can be an opening or closing wedge. A DFO is commonly performed in patients with valgus alignment of the knee, which is often caused by a deformity of the femur. On the other hand, HTO is commonly performed in patients with varus knee because in these patients the deformity is often greater at the tibia.

16.3 General Instrumentations in Osteotomies Around the Knee

- Standard instrument set for bone surgery
- Plates
- Locking Compression Plate (LCP) guide sleeve to guarantee the proper orientation of the screws
- Krackow staples can be used for high-tibial closing-wedge osteotomy
- Monocortical and bicortical locking head screws that locked at a fixed angle in a way that has no compressive effect; this allows to avoid the risk of secondary loss of correction after locking the screws
- Screwdrivers
- Several flat chisels (5–25 mm)
- Spreader chisel that allows to open the osteotomy and measure the angle of correction
- Spreaders to keep the bone gap open
- K-wires, used as guide wires bone cuts
- Sterile ruler
- Soft tissue retractors
- Screw length meter
- Oscillating saw with different sized blades [9] (Figs. 16.2 and 16.3).

Fig. 16.1 Patient position on the operating table: supine, with a tourniquet at the root of the leg

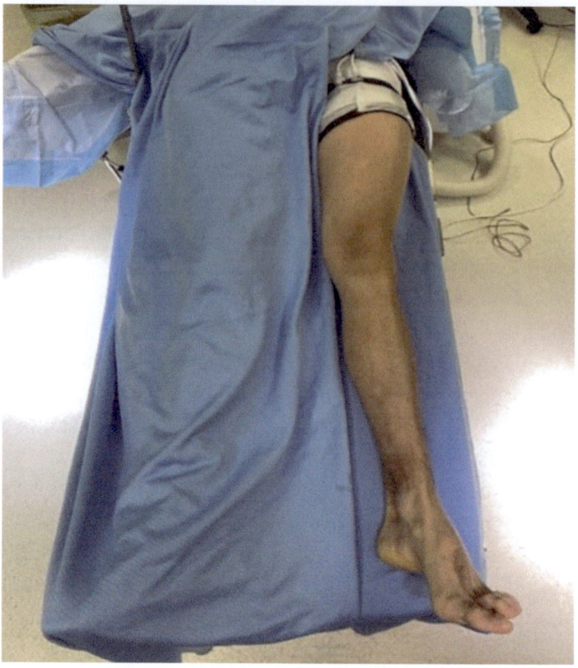

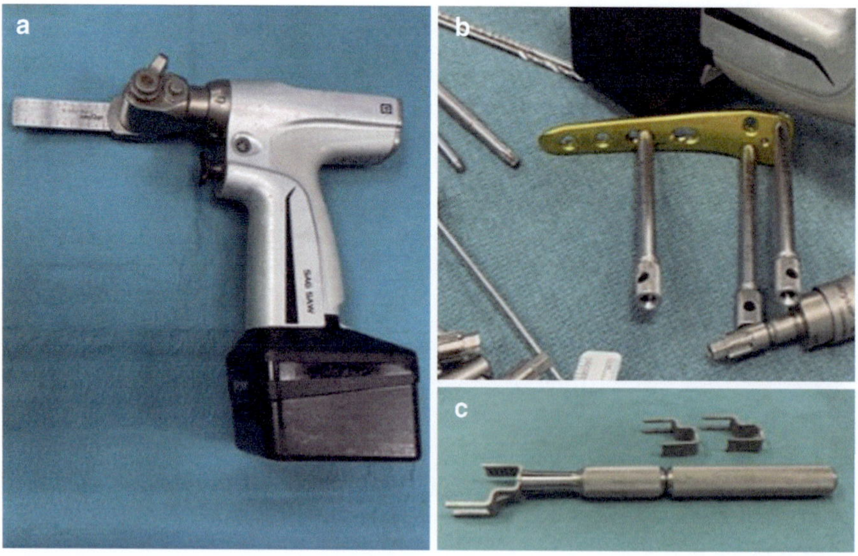

Fig. 16.3 Instruments needed for the osteotomies: (A) oscillating saw with different sized blades, (B) the TomoFix plate fixator, (C) Krakow staples

16.4 Physiological Axes of the Leg

Imaging evaluation of the patient should include anteroposterior, lateral, and 45° patellar axial views and a long double-leg standing anteroposterior alignment radiograph [7].

It is necessary to differentiate between anatomical and mechanical axes of the lower extremity. The mechanical axis is determined by drawing a line from the center of the femoral head to the center of the ankle, which corresponds to an approximately 3° incline compared with the vertical axis [7]. The mechanical axis can be subdivided into the femoral mechanical axis, which runs from the center of the femoral head to the intercondylar notch of the distal femur, and the tibial mechanical axis, which extends from the center of the proximal tibia to the center of the ankle [6].

The angle at the intersection of the femoral and the tibial mechanical axis is named hip-knee-ankle (HKA). The literature indicates a target postoperative overall leg alignment range of ±3° of neutral alignment (HKA = 180 ± 3°) (Fig. 16.1) [8].

The mechanical axis differs from the anatomical axis of the lower limb. The anatomical axes of the femur and tibia correspond to the diaphyseal midline of these long bones. However, the diaphyseal axis of the femur is not in a straight line with the anatomical axis of the tibia because of the orientation of the femoral neck [8].

The anatomical axes of the femoral and tibial diaphysis form a laterally opened angle of 173–175° anatomical femorotibial angle (aFTA) (Fig. 16.4).

Take Home Messages

1. Osteotomies aim the realignment of the mechanical axis of the lower limbs to decrease mechanical stress in the damaged compartment by transferring load into the healthy contralateral compartment.
2. Knee osteotomy can be performed by correcting the distal femur or the proximal tibia in order to establish the physiologic alignment of the whole limb.
3. Weight-bearing long AP view X-ray is essential because the mechanical axis cannot be accurately defined on standard AP X-rays of the knee.
4. The patient is positioned supine on a surgical table in order to allow full hip and knee motion during the surgery.
5. Positioning the patient in the proper way facilitates the management of correct intraoperative imaging studies, therefore the contralateral limb should be lowered and the operative one may be raised on a foam bump.

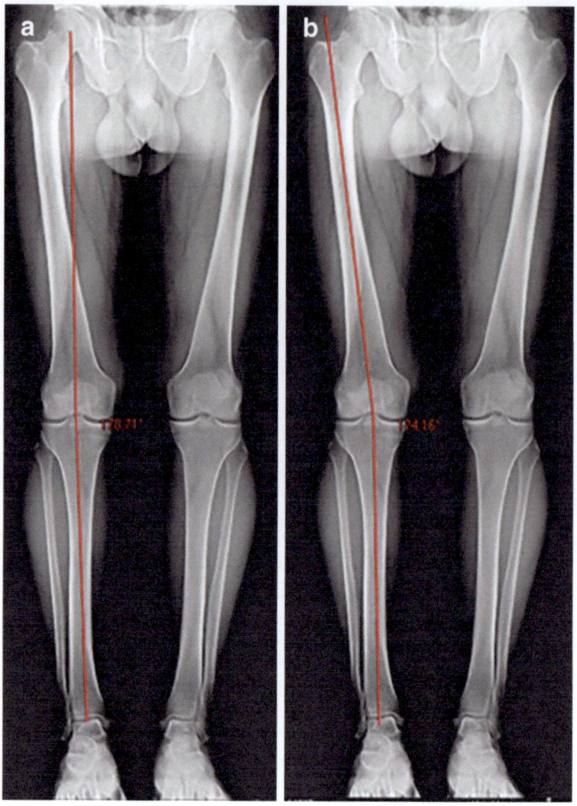

Fig. 16.4 Images of the normal mechanical and anatomic axis of the lower limb in a bilateral standing full-length anteroposterior. (**a**) HKA (hip-knee-ankle) = 180° ± 3° (178,71°). (**b**) aFTA (anatomical femorotibial angle) = laterally opened angle of 173–175° (174,16°)

References

1. Brouwer RW, Huizinga MR, Duivenvoorden T, van Raaij TM, Verhagen AP, Bierma-Zeinstra SM, Verhaar JA. Osteotomy for treating knee osteoarthritis. Cochrane Database Syst Rev. 2014;2014(12):CD004019. https://doi.org/10.1002/14651858.CD004019.pub4. PMID: 25503775; PMCID: PMC7173694.
2. Yamaguchi KT, Cheung EC, Markolf KL, et al. Effects of anterior closing wedge tibial osteotomy on anterior cruciate ligament force and knee kinematics. Am J Sports Med. 2018;46:370–7.
3. Hsu RW, Himeno S, Coventry MB, Chao EY. Normal axial alignment of the lower extremity and load-bearing distribution at the knee. Clin Orthop Relat Res. 1990;255:215–27. PMID: 2347155.
4. Peng H, Ou A, Huang X, Wang C, Wang L, Yu T, Zhang Y, Zhang Y. Osteotomy around the knee: the surgical treatment of osteoarthritis. Orthop Surg. 2021;13(5):1465–73. https://doi.org/10.1111/os.13021. Epub 2021 Jun 10. PMID: 34110088; PMCID: PMC8313165.
5. Snow M, Jermain P, Mandalia V, Murray J, Khakha R, McNicholas M, Dawson M, UK Knee Osteotomy Consensus Group. A 2021 consensus statement on osteotomies around the knee by the UK knee osteotomy consensus group (KOG). Knee. 2021;33:73–83. https://doi.org/10.1016/j.knee.2021.08.034. Epub 2021 Sep 22.. PMID: 34562741.
6. Moon HS, Choi CH, Jung M, Lee DY, Kim JH, Kim SH. The effect of knee joint rotation in the sagittal and axial plane on the measurement accuracy of coronal alignment of the lower limb.

BMC Musculoskelet Disord. 2020;21(1):470. https://doi.org/10.1186/s12891-020-03487-9. PMID: 32680484; PMCID: PMC7368736.

7. Sasaki A, Sugita T, Itaya N, Aizawa T, Miyatake N, Miyamoto S, Maeda I, Kamimura M, Takahashi A, Nagamoto H. A right angle guide for distal tuberosity osteotomy with medial open wedge high tibial osteotomy for varus knee osteoarthritis. Arthrosc Tech. 2021;10(4):e1007–16. https://doi.org/10.1016/j.eats.2020.11.017. PMID: 33981544; PMCID: PMC8084846.
8. Akiyama T, Osano K, Mizu-Uchi H, Nakamura N, Okazaki K, Nakayama H, Takeuchi R. Distal tibial tuberosity arc osteotomy in open-wedge proximal tibial osteotomy to prevent patella infra. Arthrosc Tech. 2019;8(6):e655–62. https://doi.org/10.1016/j.eats.2019.02.011. PMID: 31334025; PMCID: PMC6624185.
9. Lobenhoffer P, van Heerwaarden R, Staubli A. Osteotomies around the Knee. 1st ed. Thieme/AO; 2011. Web. 25 Sept. 2021.
10. Puddu G, Cipolla M, Cerullo G, Franco V, Giannì E. Which osteotomy for a valgus knee? Int Orthop. 2010;34(2):239–47. https://doi.org/10.1007/s00264-009-0820-3. Epub 2009 Jun 23. PMID: 19547972; PMCID: PMC2899363.
11. O'Malley MP, Pareek A, Reardon PJ, Stuart MJ, Krych AJ. Distal femoral osteotomy: lateral opening wedge technique. Arthrosc Tech. 2016;5(4):e725–30. https://doi.org/10.1016/j.eats.2016.02.037. PMID: 27709028; PMCID: PMC5039957.
12. Liu X, Chen Z, Gao Y, Zhang J, Jin Z. High tibial osteotomy: review of techniques and biomechanics. J Healthc Eng. 2019;2019:8363128. https://doi.org/10.1155/2019/8363128. PMID: 31191853; PMCID: PMC6525872.

Planning in High Tibial Osteotomy for Varus Knee

17

A. Grassi, V. Davidoni, G. Dal Fabbro, P. Agostinone, and Stefano Zaffagnini

17.1 Introduction

Osteoarthritis (OA) is the most common joint disease of adults worldwide. Its incidence rises with age. Both intrinsic and extrinsic risk factors promote its development. The knee is one of the most affected articulations by OA, especially the medial compartment [1].

Nowadays, clinically effective treatments mainly include conservative treatment, arthroplasty, and osteotomy. However, conservative treatment only offers symptomatic relief and arthroplasty is limited to patients with moderate to severe osteoarthritis. For relatively young patients who require greater knee preservation, surgical treatment with low operation trauma and a low revision rate is needed. Before the introduction of unicompartmental and total knee arthroplasty (TKA) [2], knee osteotomy was the surgical treatment of choice for medial knee OA to restore the physiologic leg alignment [3]. The advantages of osteotomy compared to TKA are the preservation of bone stock and articular proprioception, which allow high functional levels, delaying the need for joint replacement. Nowadays, many techniques are described according to the type and location of the deformity and the presence of associated lesions. Indeed, an osteotomy can be combined with articular procedures, such as anterior cruciate ligament (ACL) reconstruction, meniscal transplantation, cartilage procedures, and biological treatments, to restore normal knee biomechanics as much as possible. Hence, orthopedic surgeons should carefully evaluate all these aspects during preoperative planning, considering obtainable results from isolated or combined procedures.

The original valgus closing wedge high tibial osteotomy (CWHTO) technique performed proximal to the tuberosity was developed and diffused by Coventry in

A. Grassi (✉) · V. Davidoni · G. Dal Fabbro · P. Agostinone · S. Zaffagnini
2nd Orthopedic and Traumatologic Clinic, IRCCS Istituto Ortopedico Rizzoli, Bologna, Italy
e-mail: alberto.grassi@ior.it

G. M. Marcheggiani Muccioli et al. (eds.), *Easy Planning in Elective Primary Orthopedic Procedures*, https://doi.org/10.1007/978-3-031-77006-7_17

1965 [3, 4]. For a considerable time, the closing wedge procedure was a widespread method in treating medial knee osteoarthritis until the open-wedge technique gained new popularity. This development was promoted by the introduction of new implant designs, especially plates with angular stable locking head screws ("internal fixators") during the last years [5]. The medial opening wedge technique with these implants offers many advantages.

The main features and planning of OWHTO and CWHTO are described in this chapter.

17.2 Varus Knee

Lower limb axes can be pathologically altered in the frontal, sagittal, and/or transverse plane.

On the frontal plane, the main axis that the surgeon should consider are the mechanical axis (Mikulicz line or weight-bearing line, WBL) passing through the Fujisawa point, located at 62% [6] across the width of the tibial plateau from medial to lateral, mechanical axis deviation (MAD), hip-knee-ankle (HKA), medial proximal tibial angle (MPTA), lateral distal femoral angle (LDFA), and joint line convergence angle (JLCA) (Fig. 17.1a and 17.1b).

The posterior tibial slope and patellar height should be carefully evaluated on the sagittal plane. Furthermore, wear due to anterior tibial subluxation can be associated with ACL lesion. Stress radiographs may be helpful to assess latent soft tissue laxity of the collateral knee ligaments. Latent soft tissue laxity is defined as the amount of soft tissue that can be extended to valgus or varus from the weight-bearing position, and it is calculated by subtracting the JLCA on weight-bearing standing radiographs from that on stress radiograph. The JLCA change could be larger in patients with significant latent medial laxity or severe varus deformity requiring a large correction, which could lead to unexpected overcorrection in high tibial osteotomy (HTO). Thus, postoperative JLCA change should be considered in preoperative surgical planning. Target point shifting within the Fujisawa point could be a strategy to prevent overcorrection, especially in patients with considerable latent medial laxity [7, 8].

Another critical factor to consider is the location of the deformity, which can be intra-articular or extra-articular. This aspect influences the site of the osteotomy. Indeed, deformity correction should be performed at its source (femur, tibia, or both) and, if possible, at the center of rotation of angulation (CORA). CORA is the angle formed between the intersection of the proximal and distal axis of a deformed bone and it is a measure of the angular deformity. If the osteotomy line passes through CORA, realignment occurs without translation. When the osteotomy is performed at another level than at the CORA, the axis will not only realign by angulation but translation will occur as well. In that case, correction of the mechanical axis may be achieved but a pathological joint line orientation may be the secondary adverse result.

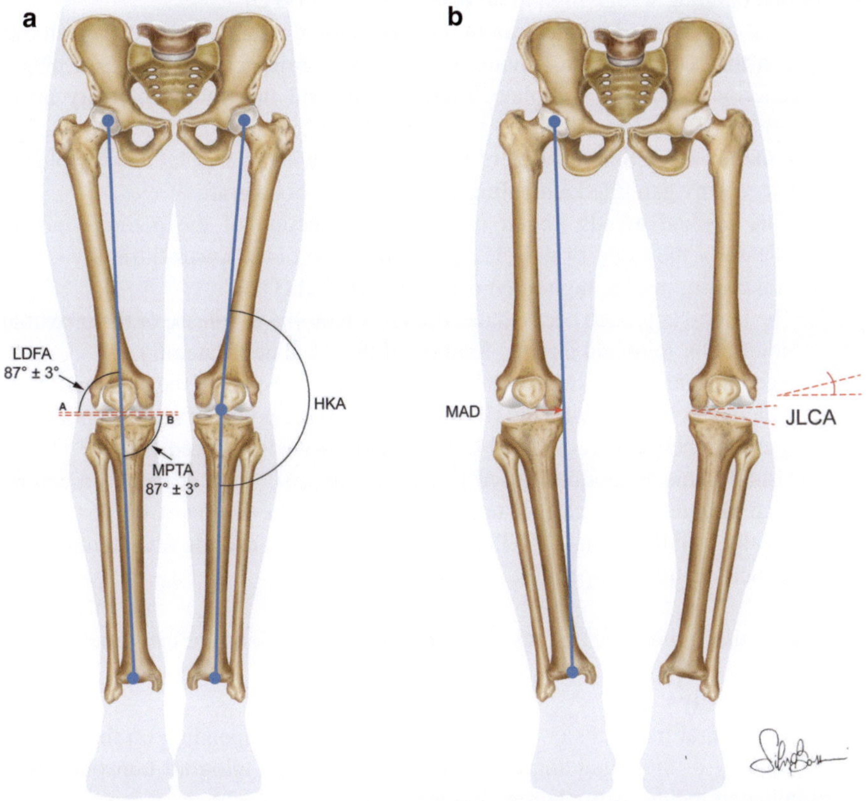

Fig. 17.1 (**a** and **b**) Main axes of the lower limb on the frontal plane: (**a**) on the right leg is represented Mikulicz line (or weight-bearing line, WBL) passing through the Fujisawa point, medial proximal tibial angle (MPTA) = 87° ± 3° and lateral distal femoral angle (LDFA) = 87° ± 3°, on the left leg is represented the hip-knee-ankle (HKA); (**b**) on the right leg is represented mechanical axis deviation (MAD) and joint line convergence angle (JLCA) on the left one. Copyright of Silvia Bassini, 2024. All rights reserved

Usually, medial compartment overload caused by varus malalignment can be corrected with osteotomies of the proximal tibia, including medial opening wedge (OWHTO) and lateral closing wedge (CWHTO) procedures. Valgus malalignment is typically addressed with osteotomies of the distal femur and will be described in another chapter.

17.3 Types of HTO

Two different surgical techniques are used to restore the mechanical axes as mentioned above:

- Medial opening wedge high tibial osteotomy (OWHTO):
  1. Performed as a biplanar osteotomy: horizontal osteotomy of the posterior two-thirds of the tibia leaving a lateral bone bridge of 10 mm as a hinge; anterior ascending complete osteotomy behind the tibial tuberosity at an angle of 110°. The osteotomy is opened slowly, ensuring that the lateral hinge remains intact. Stabilization of the correction with an angular locking plate.
  2. Osteotomy gap filled with allograft cancellous bone graft.
  3. This method avoids fibular osteotomy, dissection of the peroneal nerve, release of the extensor muscles, and shortening of the lower extremity.
- Lateral closing wedge high tibial osteotomy (CWHTO):
  1. The lateral approach necessitates fibular osteotomy or release of the proximal tibiofibular joint and internal fixation of the tibial head laterally.
  2. Need to detach the extensor muscles at the lateral aspect of the proximal tibia, which is associated with the risk of damage to the peroneal nerve, reported in literature between 3.3% and 11.9% for closed-wedge procedures [9].
  3. Usually, this technique is used to perform an associated articular procedure such as anterior cruciate ligament reconstruction/revision (ACLR) or meniscal allograft transplant (MAT) to avoid screws when drilling tibial tunnels and reduce the tibial slope [10].

In general, for both techniques, the main contraindications are the same:

- Severe obesity
- Loss of lateral meniscus or loss of medial meniscus, depending on the amount and quality of the remaining tissue (consider meniscal allograft transplantation or collagen meniscus implant within HTO)
- Severe degenerative joint disease, second- or third-degree cartilage damage in the lateral compartment according to the Kellgren–Lawrence classification
- Limited range of motion at the knee joint, especially extension deficits >10°
- Poor soft-tissue condition at the proximal tibial
- Local acute or chronic inflammation

In Fig. 17.2 the main differences between the two techniques are summarized.

17.4 Planning in HTO

Preoperative planning should be done on a full-length anteroposterior radiograph with double-leg standing and posteroanterior views in 45° of flexion (Rosenberg view) and lateral views.

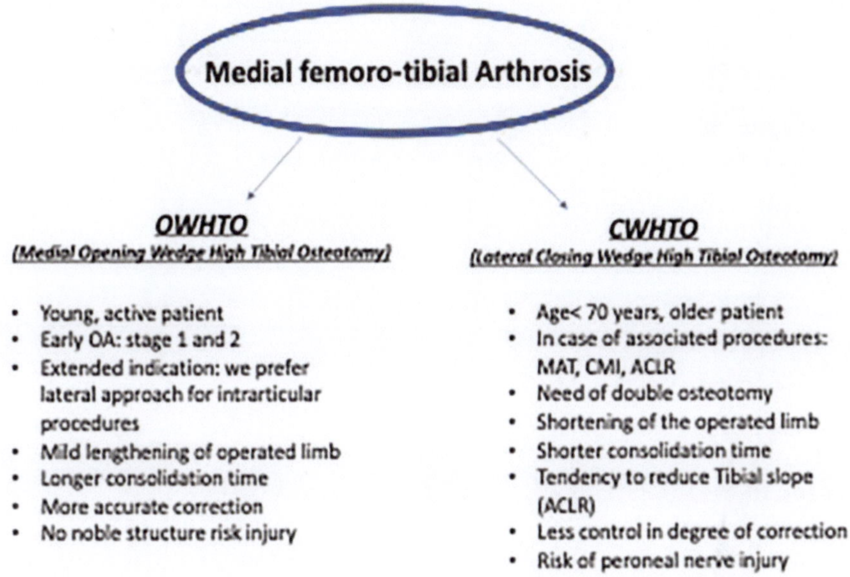

Fig. 17.2 Summary of the main features of OWHTO and CWHTO

17.5 Planning: The Miniaci Method

The degree of correction is calculated with the method described by Miniaci et al. [11]. Miniaci et al. recommend using the WBL to determine the coronal plane correction. The hinge of osteotomy is considered the starting point for correction α angle measurement. The correction angle is included between a line passing through the center of the ankle joint and a line passing to the distal apex of the correct mechanical axis. The angle formed by those two lines is the planned correction angle.

In closing wedge osteotomies, the hinge point is located in the medial proximal tibial metaphysis, approximately 2.5 cm below the joint line. In an opening wedge osteotomy, this hinge projects onto the lateral proximal metaphysis on the level of the proximal border of the tibiofibular joint, around 15 mm below the subchondral sclerosis zone of the lateral plateau. This angle can now be drawn on the proximal tibia using the defined hinge point as the tip of the triangle. In a closing wedge osteotomy, the two planes of the osteotomy are marked and the base of the triangle on the lateral cortex corresponds to the height of the wedge to be resected (Fig. 17.3). In an opening wedge osteotomy, the triangle should also be drawn and the base of the triangle on the medial cortex corresponds the opening degrees of the osteotomy (Fig. 17.4). The defect created by the saw blade must be considered when the surgery is done.

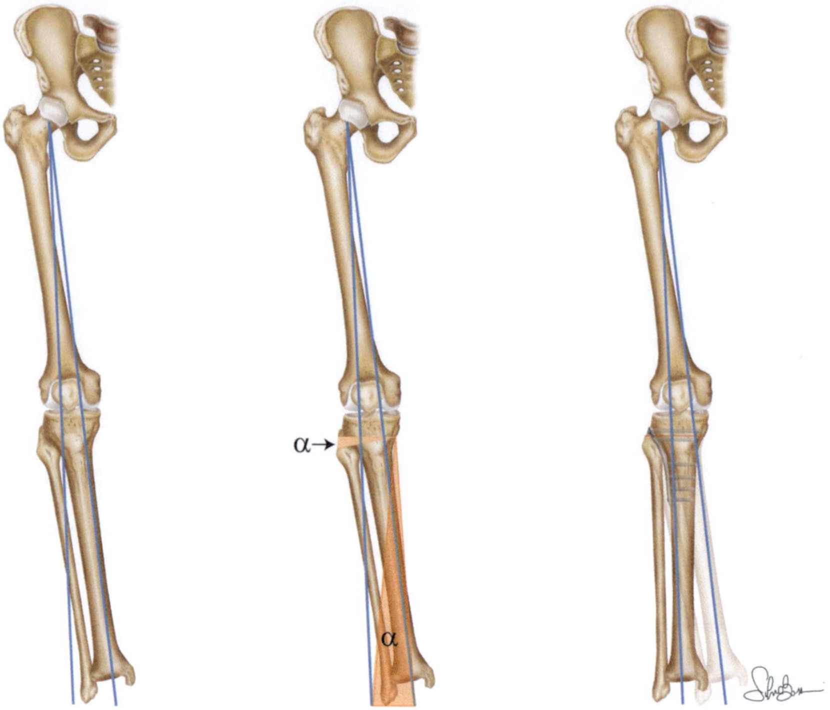

Fig. 17.3 The hinge of planned osteotomy is considered as starting point for correction angle measurement. The correction angle (α) is included between a line passing through the center of the ankle joint and a line passing to the distal apex of the correct mechanical axis. Copyright of Silvia Bassini, 2024. All rights reserved

17.6 Planning: The Dugdale Method

Dugdale et al. [12] use the WBL for preoperative planning and have described two planning methods. In the first method, the first line is drawn from the center of the femoral head to 62% of the tibial width from medial to lateral. The second line is drawn from the center of the tibiotalar joint to the 62% coordinate. The angle formed by these two lines is the correction angle (Fig. 17.5). In the second planning method, a line is drawn from the center of the hip to the 62% coordinate, the X-ray is cut in line with the osteotomy side and the distal tibia is rotated until the WBL passes through the 62% coordinate. The correction angle corresponds to the lateral overlap for lateral closed-wedge osteotomies or the medial opening for medial open-wedge osteotomies.

Since both suggested planning methods arrive at equivalent correction angles, all methods are equally suitable [13].

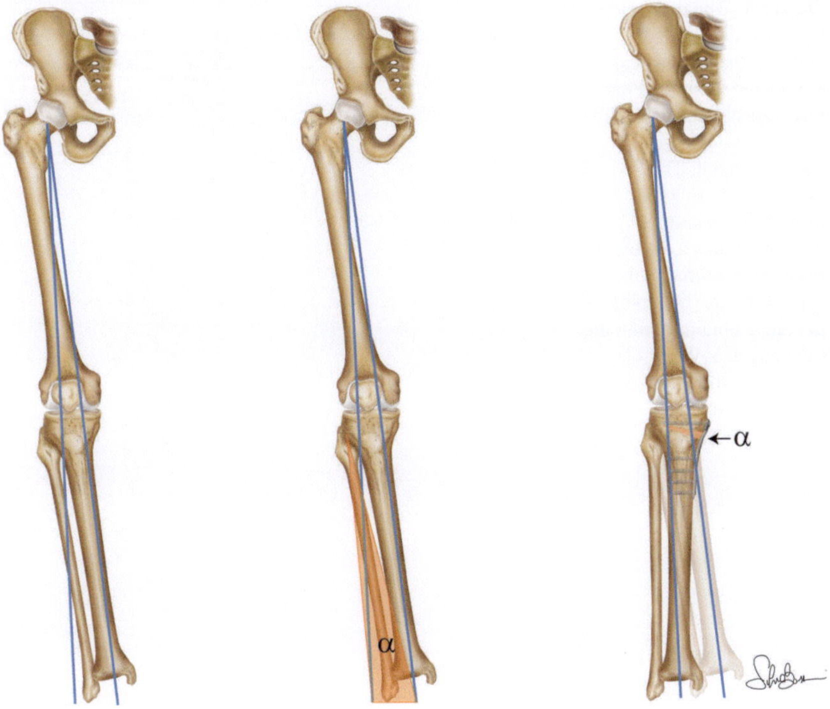

Fig. 17.4 The hinge of planned osteotomy is considered as starting point for correction angle measurement. The correction angle (α) is included between a line passing through the center of the ankle joint and a line passing to the distal apex of the correct mechanical axis.

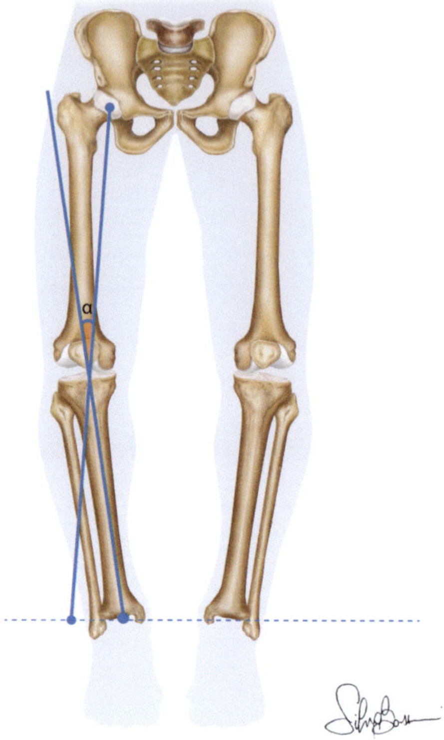

Fig. 17.5 The correction angle (α) is included between the mechanical axis of the femur and the mechanical axis of the tibia passing through the Fujisawa point. The amount of bone to be resected to obtain the desired angular correction must bc measured at the osteotomy site by reporting the angle obtained from the planning.

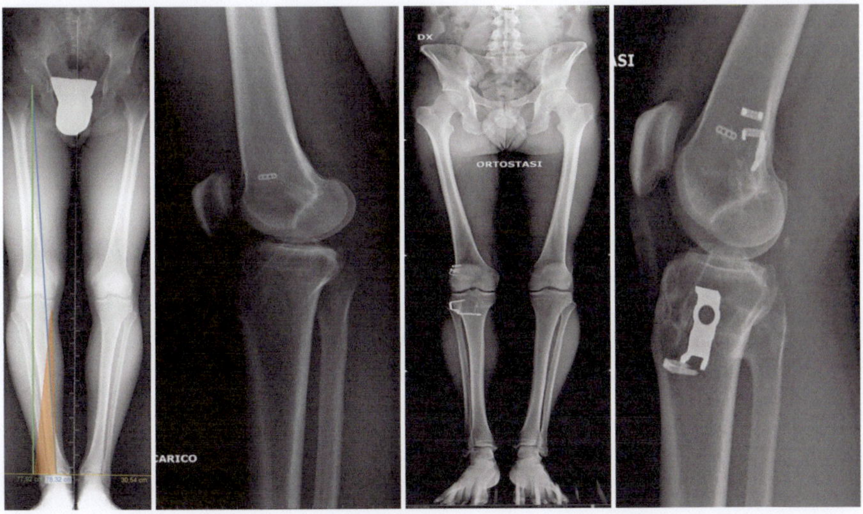

OWHTO: Pre- and post-op panoramic and lateral X-rays

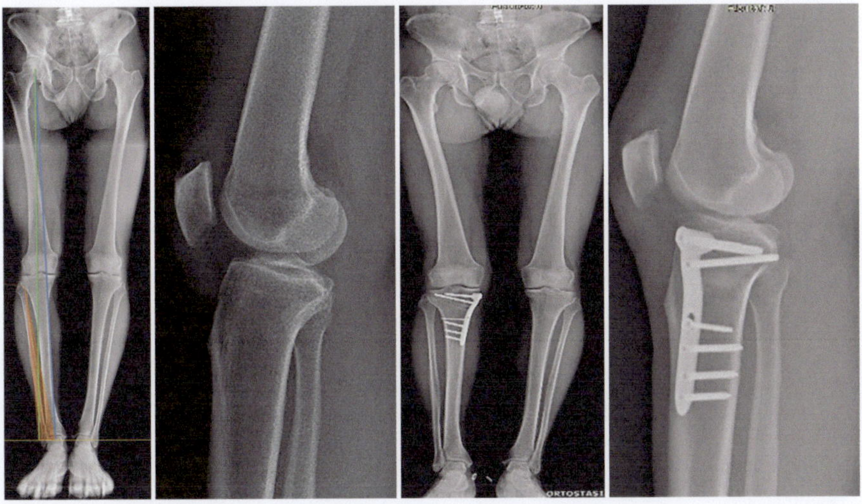

CWHTO: Pre- and post-op panoramic and lateral X-rays

Take Home Messages

1. Osteotomy represents a reliable and effective technique to restore the physiologic limb axes and delay medial articular degeneration.
2. It is a biological, safe, joint-sparing, and cost-effective surgery.

3. The goal of surgery is to recreate neutral alignment or overcorrect the WBL, the mechanical axis line has to pass through the center or the lateral part of the knee, depending on surgeon planning.
4. To calculate the amount of correction needed, preoperative planning is required to achieve the target accurately.
5. OWHTO is more accurate for the correction of the deformity, needs a longer time to consolidate, and may result in mild limb lengthening.
6. CWHTO is less accurate for the correction, needs a shorter time to consolidate, and may result in limb shortening.
7. Both techniques are associable with intra-articular procedures but CWHTO is recommended for the lateral approach and the tendency to decrease tibial slope (in particular, in ACL revision).

References

1. Michael JW-P, Schlüter-Brust KU, Eysel P. The epidemiology, etiology, diagnosis, and treatment of osteoarthritis of the knee. Dtsch Arztebl Int. 2010;107(9):152–62.
2. Diduch DR, Insall JN, Scott WN, et al. Total knee replacement in young, active patients. Long-term follow-up and functional outcome. J Bone Joint Surg Am. 1997;79:575–82.
3. Coventry MB. Osteotomy of the upper portion of the tibia for degenerative arthritis of the knee. A preliminary report. J Bone Joint Surg Am. 1965;47:984–90.
4. Coventry MB. Upper tibial osteotomy for osteoarthritis. J Bone Joint Surg Am. 1985;67(7):1136–40.
5. Franco V, Cerullo G, Cipolla M, et al. Open wedge high tibial osteotomy. Tech Knee Surg. 2002;1(1):43–53.
6. Fujisawa Y, Masuhara K, Shiomi S. The effect of high tibial osteotomy on osteoarthritis of the knee. An arthroscopic study of 54 knee joints. Orthop Clin North Am 1979;10:585–608.
7. Paley D, Pfeil J. Principles of deformity corrections around the knee. Orthopade. 2000;29(1):18–38.
8. Lee DK, Wang JH, Won Y, Min YK, Jaiswal S, Lee BH, et al. Preoperative latent medial laxity and correction angle are crucial factors for overcorrection in medial open-wedge high tibial osteotomy. Knee Surg Sports Traumatol Arthrosc Off J ESSKA. 2020;28:1411–8.
9. Coventry MB. Upper tibial osteotomy. Clin Orthop Relat Res. 1984;182:46–52.
10. Yamaguchi KT, Cheung EC, Markolf KL, et al. Effects of anterior closing wedge tibial osteotomy on anterior cruciate ligament force and knee kinematics. Am J Sports Med. 2018;46:370–7.
11. Miniaci A, Ballmer FT, Ballmer PM, et al. Proximal tibial osteotomy. A new fixation device. Clin Orthop Relat Res. 1989;246:250–9.
12. Dugdale TW, Noyes FR, Styer D. Preoperative planning for high tibial osteotomy. The effect of lateral tibiofemoral separation and tibiofemoral length. Clin Orthop Relat Res. 1992;274:248–64.
13. Brown G, Amendola A. Radiographic evaluation and preoperative planning for high tibial osteotomies. Operative Techn Sports Med. 2000;8:2–14.

Planning in Distal Femoral Osteotomy for Valgus Knee

18

A. Grassi, P. Agostinone, G. Dal Fabbro, G. A. Lucidi, A. Pagano, and Stefano Zaffagnini

18.1 Introduction

The mechanical alignment of the lower limb is a critical factor in the genesis and progression of knee osteoarthritis (OA) [1, 8]. Patients with valgus malalignment are predisposed to increased wear of the lateral femoro-tibial compartment, with a five-fold increase in the odds of lateral OA progression [1]. Distal femoral osteotomy (DFO) is a surgical option to correct the valgus malalignment through a medial shift of the mechanical axis. DFO can be accomplished via a lateral opening wedge (LOW-DFO) or medial closing wedge (MCW-DFO) technique. This technique is a joint-sparing procedure aiming to delay knee arthroplasty. Several clinical studies showed the importance of the correct indication and patient selection to achieve long-term satisfactory clinical results [9, 12]. Distal femoral varus-producing osteotomy can be performed in the lateral meniscal allograft transplant (LMAT) setting to correct valgus malalignment of the knee and thus offload the lateral compartment [2].

In this chapter, we will describe the planning of the operative technique for a lateral opening wedge and [13] a medial closing wedge varus-producing distal femoral osteotomy.

A. Grassi (✉) · P. Agostinone · G. Dal Fabbro · G. A. Lucidi · A. Pagano · S. Zaffagnini
2nd Orthopedic and Traumatologic Clinic, IRCCS Istituto Ortopedico Rizzoli, Bologna, Italy
e-mail: alberto.grassi@ior.it

G. M. Marcheggiani Muccioli et al. (eds.), *Easy Planning in Elective Primary Orthopedic Procedures*, https://doi.org/10.1007/978-3-031-77006-7_18

18.2 Valgus Knee

In valgus malalignment of the lower extremity, the anatomical femorotibial angle (aFTA) is less than 173–175°. In relevant valgus deformity, the mechanical axis distance from the knee joint's center is larger than 10 mm [6], and the distance between the medial malleoli is increased.

Other authors consider valgus malalignment when the mechanical axis lies lateral to the tip of the lateral tibial eminence or more than 56% from the medial edge of the tibial plateau in thc coronal plane (Fig. 18.1) [5].

18.3 Planning

The goal of surgery is to recreate neutral alignment, such that the mechanical axis line passes through the center of the knee. For optimal correction, the osteotomy should be performed at the apex of the deformity to restore the physiological axes.

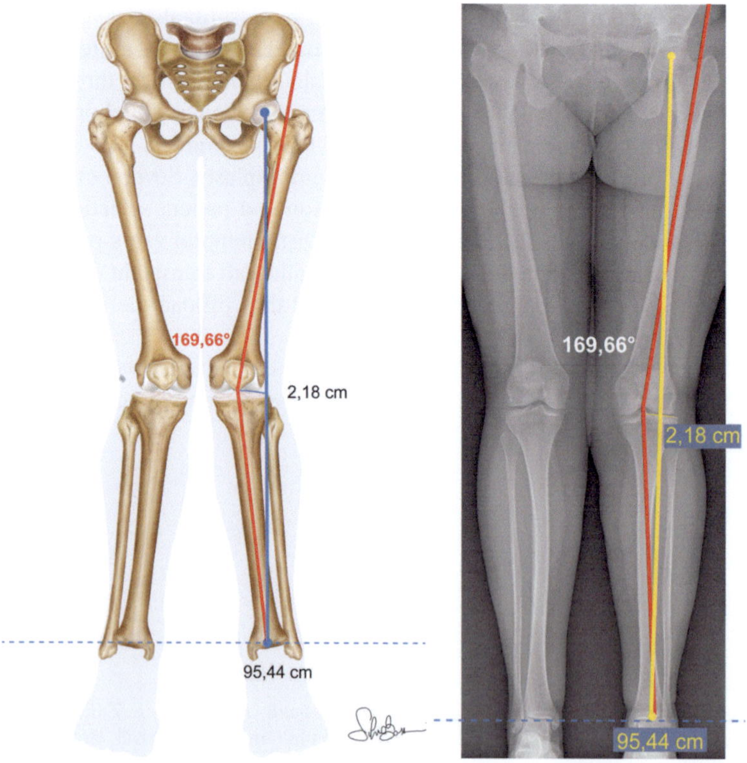

Fig. 18.1 Images of the valgus malalignment of the left knee. aFTA is laterally opened angle of 169,66°. The mechanical axis distance from the knee joint's center is 2.18 cm.

In patients with valgus deformity associated with lateral compartment osteoarthritis, the corrected mechanical axis can be planned at 0–20% medially in relation to the center of the tibia, depending on cartilage loss [4].

18.4 Opening Wedge DFO

To calculate the amount of opening, the surgeon calculates the correction angle (Fig. 18.2):

- A point located at 50% of the tibial width (between the medial and lateral tibial eminence) is marked on the AP view of the long leg radiograph.
- Two lines are drawn connecting this point with the center of the femoral head and the center of the ankle joint (femoral mechanical axis and the tibial mechanical axis).
- The acute angle joining the extension of these two lines is the angle of correction.

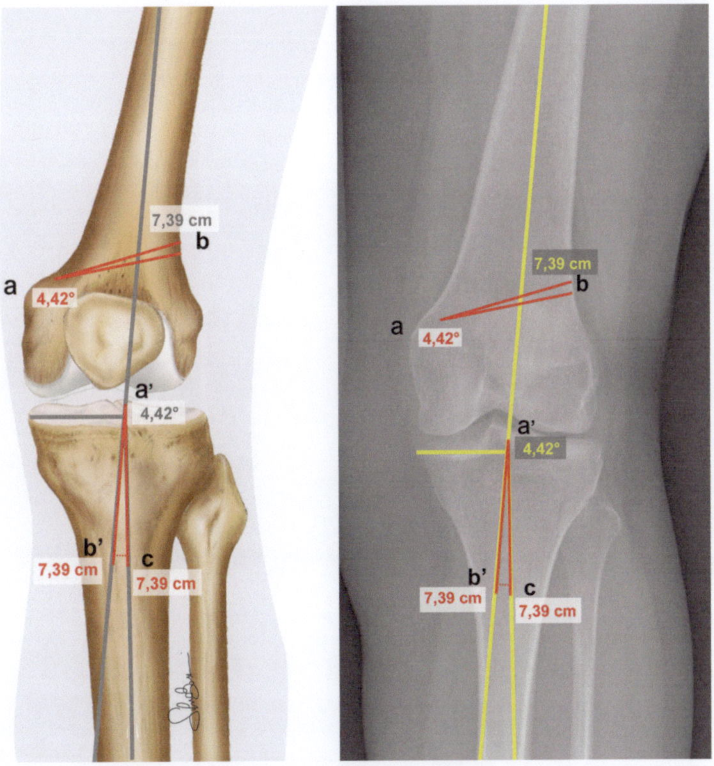

Fig. 18.2 Image and radiographic planning of opening wedge DFO.

- Then the osteotomy line is drawn: this should be oriented from lateral to medial (ending close to the adductor tubercle) and proximal to distal (20° with respect to the axis perpendicular to the femoral shaft) (ab).
- The length of the osteotomy is measured, and this distance is transferred on both rays of the angle of correction starting from the apex (a'b' and a'c). The base of the isosceles triangle (b'c) obtained in this fashion is the opening required at the osteotomy [7].

It is essential that the hinge position is between 0.5 and 1 cm apart to avoid hinge fractures in lateral open wedge [10].

18.5 Closing Wedge DFO

To calculate the amount of the closure, the surgeon calculates the angle of correction (Fig. 18.3):

- The mechanical axis passes through the lateral compartment of the knee (A–D).

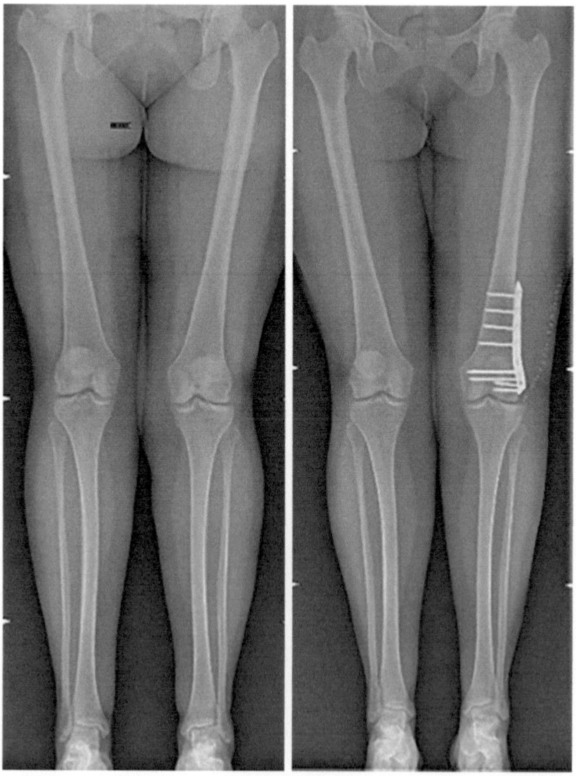

Fig. 18.3 Image of pre- and post-surgery

- A line is drawn from the center of the tibial plateau (A) through just medial to the medial tibial spine (C) to create a new desired and mechanical axis line. This line is prolonged to a level of the femoral head (E).
- A hinge point (H) is detected at the lateral cortex of the supracondylar region, considering 0.5–1 cm from the cortical to avoid hinge fractures.
- An expected correctional angle (α) is measured at this level between two lines: one line is drawn from the center of the femoral head (D) to the hinge point and the other line is drawn from the hinge point to point E.
- The angle α is the angle of correction.
- Correction angle α is projected at the distal femur using two oblique down sloping lines of equal length converging at the hinge point.
- The distance measured between those two lines at the level of the medial cortex represents the osteotomy wedge base length to be removed during surgery [3, 11] (Figs. 18.4 and 18.5).

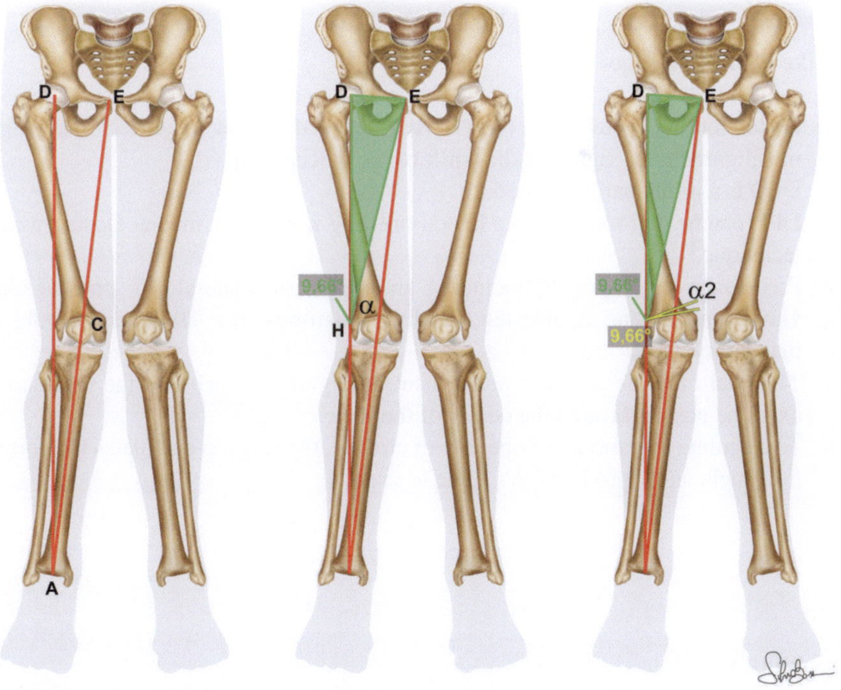

Fig. 18.4 Image of closing wedge DFO planning.

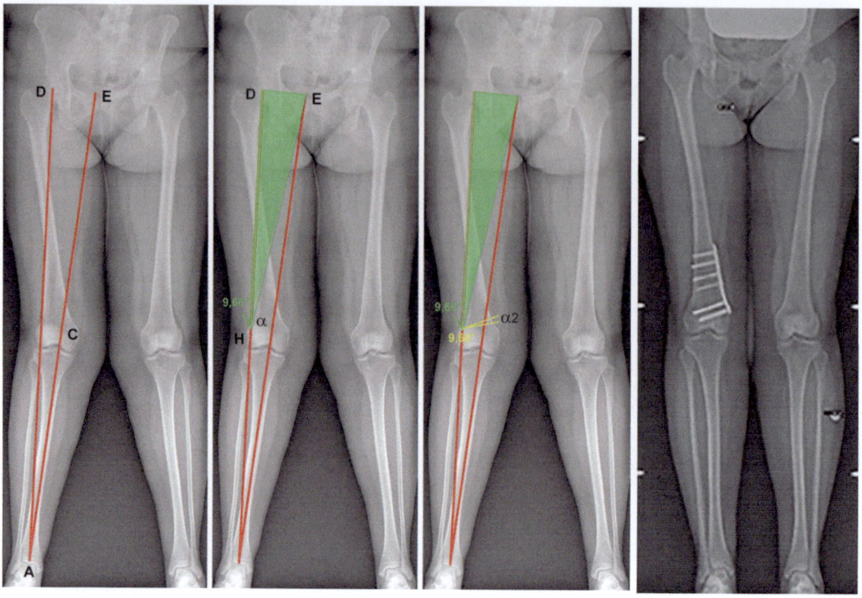

Fig. 18.5 Radiographic image of closing wedge DFO planning and postoperative radiograph after DFO

Take Home Messages

1. Distal femoral osteotomy (DFO) is a surgical option to correct the valgus malalignment through a medial shift of the mechanical axis.
2. DFO is a joint-sparing procedure.
3. DFO can be performed with a lateral opening wedge or a medial closing wedge technique.
4. Preoperative radiographs, including anteroposterior, lateral, 45° patellar axial views, and a long double-leg standing anteroposterior alignment should be mandatory.
5. The goal of surgery is to recreate neutral alignment, such that the mechanical axis line passes through the center of the knee.
6. To calculate the amount of opening or closing, the surgeon calculates the correction angle and reproduces the angle in vivo.

References

1. Haddad FS, Bentley G. Total knee arthroplasty after high tibial osteotomy: a medium-term review. J Arthroplast. 2000;15(5):597–603.
2. Harris JD, Hussey K, Saltzman BM, McCormick FM, Wilson H, Abrams GD, Cole BJ. Cartilage repair with or without meniscal transplantation and osteotomy for lateral compartment chondral defects of the knee: case series with minimum 2-year follow-up. Orthop J Sports Med. 2014;2(10):2325967114551528.
3. Van Heerwaarden R, Brinkman J-M, Pronk Y. Correction of femoral valgus deformity. J Knee Surg. 2017;30(8):746–55.
4. Johnson F, Leitl S, Waugh W. The distribution of load across the knee. A comparison of static and dynamic measurements. J Bone Joint Surg Br. 1980;62(3):346–9.
5. Laprade RF, Spiridonov SI, Nystrom LM, Jansson KS. Prospective outcomes of young and middle-aged adults with medial compartment osteoarthritis treated with a proximal tibial opening wedge osteotomy. Arthroscopy. 2012;28(3):354–64.
6. Paley D, Pfeil J. Principles of deformity correction around the knee. Orthopade. 2000;29(1):18–38.
7. Pilone C, Rosso F, Cottino U, Rossi R, Bonasia DE. Lateral opening wedge distal femoral osteotomy for lateral compartment arthrosis/overload. Clin Sports Med. 2019;38(3):351–9.
8. Sharma L, Song J, Felson DT, Cahue S, Shamiyeh E, Dunlop DD. The role of knee alignment in disease progression and functional decline in knee osteoarthritis. JAMA. 2001;286(2):188–95.
9. Weidow J. Lateral osteoarthritis of the knee. Etiology based on morphological, anatomical, kinematic and kinetic observations. Acta Orthop Suppl. 2006;77(322):3–44.
10. Winkler PW, Rupp MC, Lutz PM, Geyer S, Forkel P, Imhoff AB, Feucht MJ. A hinge position distal to the adductor tubercle minimizes the risk of hinge fractures in lateral open wedge distal femoral osteotomy. Knee Surg Sports Traumatol Arthrosc. 2021;29(10):3382–91.
11. Yoo JD, Kim NK. Distal femoral varization osteotomy. J Korean Orthop Assoc. 2014;49(2):118–25.
12. Yusuf E, Bijsterbosch J, Slagboom PE, Rosendaal FR, Huizinga TWJ, Kloppenburg M. Body mass index and alignment and their interaction as risk factors for progression of knees with radiographic signs of osteoarthritis. Osteoarthr Cartil. 2011;19(9):1117–22.
13. Zaffagnini S, Marcheggiani Muccioli GM, Grassi A, Roberti di Sarsina T, Raggi F, Signorelli C, Urrizola F, Spinnato P, Rimondi E, Marcacci M. Over-the-top ACL reconstruction plus extra-articular lateral tenodesis with hamstring tendon grafts: prospective evaluation with 20-year minimum follow-up. Am J Sports Med. 2017;45(14):3233–42.

Part VII

Ankle Arthroplasty

M. Mosca

19 Patient Positioning and Planning in Total Ankle Replacement Through Anterior and Lateral Approach

S. Caravelli, M. Viotto, G. Puccetti, A. Baiardi, M. Di Ponte, B. Khateeb, and M. Mosca

19.1 Introduction

Ankle osteoarthritis (AO) is one of the leading causes of chronic disability in an increasing part of the world's population [1]. The first therapeutic choice is conservative management, but in case of lack of improvement of the symptoms, surgical treatment should be taken into consideration. The indications for total ankle replacement in the last years are increased, thanks to advances in surgical technique, materials, and design [2]. Due to the improvement of total ankle implants in the 1970s, total ankle replacements (TAR) have increased in frequency as an alternative treatment option to arthrodesis.

The most common way to perform a TAR is via a direct anterior approach through the interval between the tibialis anterior and extensor hallucis longus tendons [3].

The main objective of this chapter is to illuminate preoperative planning techniques for ankle prostheses through anterior access. In these few pages, the authors want to emphasize how the study of the patient through the clinic and diagnostic examinations allows the orthopedist to arrive as prepared as possible for surgery for the best outcome for the surgeon and patient.

S. Caravelli · G. Puccetti · A. Baiardi · M. Di Ponte · B. Khateeb · M. Mosca (✉)
Bentivoglio Orthopaedic Unit, IRCCS Istituto Ortopedico Rizzoli, Bologna, Italy
e-mail: massimiliano.mosca@ior.it

M. Viotto
IRCCS Istituto Ortopedico Rizzoli, S.C. Ortopedia Pediatria, Bologna, Italy

G. M. Marcheggiani Muccioli et al. (eds.), *Easy Planning in Elective Primary Orthopedic Procedures*, https://doi.org/10.1007/978-3-031-77006-7_19

19.2 Positioning

The positioning of the patient is of fundamental importance in every surgical procedure, especially in the orthopedic surgery of the lower limb. A patient well-placed on the operating table will allow the surgeon and the assistants to focus their attention on the procedure, while incorrect or unstable positioning will make the surgery more difficult.

In ankle prosthetic surgery, the patient's positioning is necessarily "suggested" by the instruments used and by the surgical approach.

In anteriorly implanted prosthetic design, the entire procedure is performed with the patient in supine decubitus, limb tending to intra-rotation (we suggest inserting a gel pillow below the homolateral buttock), and foot slightly outside the operating table in order to allow free plantarflexion and dorsiflexion.

In the case of laterally implanted ankle components (currently, only a prosthetic model requires this approach), the patient is first placed on the contralateral side of the affected limb in order to have a direct vision of the operating field and surgical approach. The first surgical step involves a distal tilting osteotomy of the fibula to have direct lateral access to the tibiotalar joint. Then the patient is placed in the supine decubitus to perform the guided bone resections and the position of the definitive components.

19.3 Planning

The first step for correct planning of a TAR is to perform a *physical examination* that includes careful inspection of the foot and ankle while walking and standing with special attention given to obvious deformities and skin and soft tissue condition. It is also important to assess the alignment of the ankle and hindfoot, the degree of instability and reducibility of the deformity, tightness of the Achilles tendon, and forefoot pronation with a careful physical examination (Fig. 19.1) [4].

To properly plan a TAR, it is necessary to get a weight-bearing anteroposterior (AP) and lateral *conventional radiographic study* of the ankle. Saltzman's view should be used to assess the infra malleolar alignment. This radiographic projection is taken by positioning the patient with feet parallel and knees extended, under load. The X-ray tube is oriented 20° from the horizontal and placed near the patient (Fig. 19.2) [5].

The supramalleolar ankle alignment should be evaluated in the coronal plane by measurement of the medial distal tibial angle and sagittal plane by measurement of the anterior distal tibial angle (Figs. 19.3 and 19.4) [6].

MRI imaging is often indicated to get additional information when associated soft tissue pathology, such as a peroneal or posterior tibialis tendon tear, is suspected. Some authors reported that 3D templating with an *MRI or CT* scan is significantly more accurate than using an AP X-ray [7]. Other authors do not recommend the routine use of magnetic resonance imaging in patients with ankle OA, but they advise to use a single-photon-emission computed tomography (*SPECT-CT scan*) in

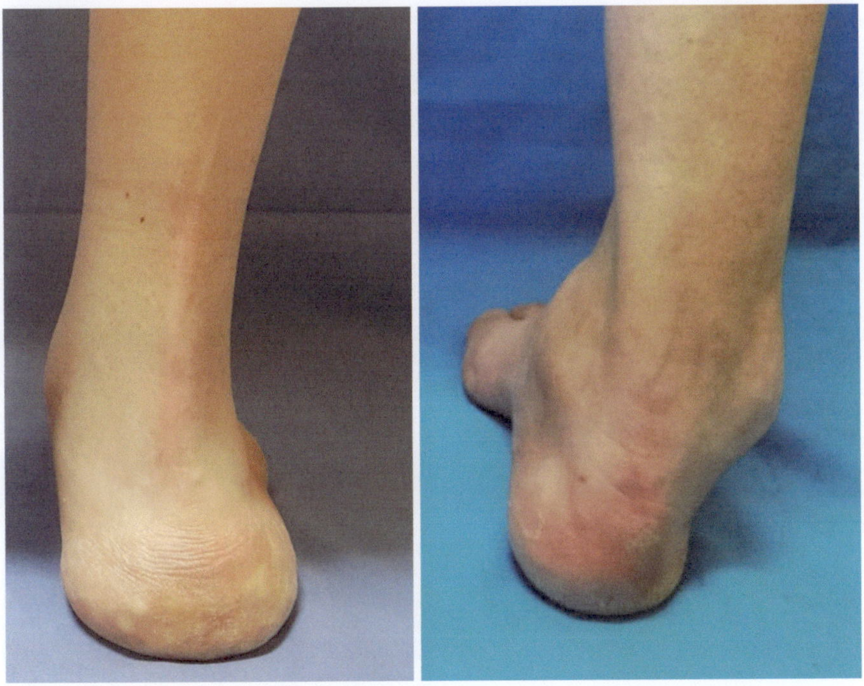

Fig. 19.1 Clinical image of valgus (left side) and varus (right side) ankle–hindfoot

patients with degenerative changes of the adjacent joints to evaluate the morphologic changes and biological activities [4].

A tool that can help surgeons to be more and more accurate in complicated ankle joint replacement is computer-assisted surgery (*CAS*), a technique that relies on computer assistance and 3D images for pre-surgical planning. The multimedia system allows us to obtain better surgical and clinical results [8, 9].

It is necessary to evaluate instability and malalignment with these preoperative exams during the planning because both can cause edge-loading and sub-dislocation of the liner, progressive deformity and high rate of early failure. To consider the ankle alignment in the coronal plane, a standing AP X-ray is used to measure the angle between the anatomical axis of the tibia and a line perpendicular to the articular surface of the talus dome. An ankle is regarded as neutral if the degrees of alignment are less than 10° of varus or valgus; on the other hand, if the degrees of alignment are more than 10°, the ankle is labeled as varus and requires corrective osteotomy at the level of deformity [6]. In varus ankles, it is essential to calculate, always on the AP standing X-ray, the angle between the tibial plafond and the talar dome, called the talar tilt. If the talar tilt is more than 10°, the joint is considered incongruent and a release of the medial contracted ligamentous structures should move the tilted talus parallel to the neutral plafond, making the ankle neutral. On the other hand, if the talar tilt is less than 10°, the deformity is called congruent and a neutralizing tibia cut should follow the medial release [6].

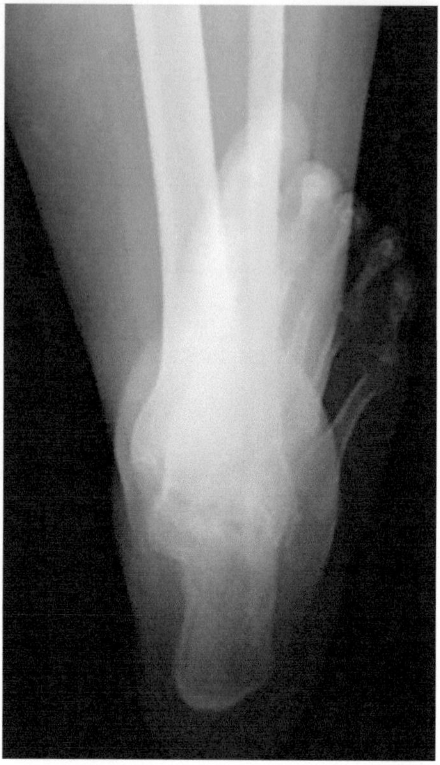

Fig. 19.2 Saltzman view X-ray

In case of sagittal deformities, such as an anteposition of the talar dome or altered inclination of the tibial plafond, these require correction to allow the restoration of the original center of rotation. In the case of talar anteposition with respect to the tibia (sometimes a consequence of severe chronic ankle instabilities), the distal tibial slope (β angle) [10] needs to be corrected by a tibial resection that allows to have a tibial plafond parallel to the ground, or in case of severe astragal anteposition, a few degrees inverse tibial slope can be a proper alignment in the experience of the authors (Fig. 19.5).

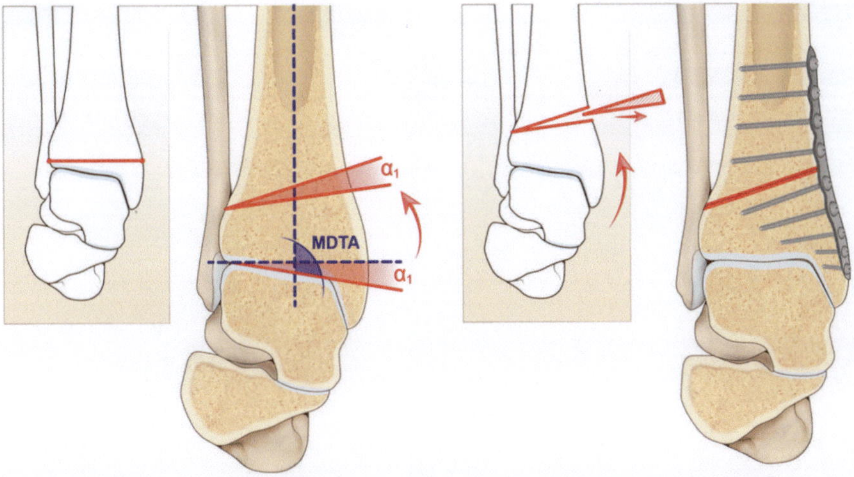

Fig. 19.3 Visual artwork showing alfa angle of correction and MDTA (medial distal tibia angle). A supramelleolar osteotomy can be considered as an accessory procedure during total ankle replacement in case of severe ankle varus or valgus deformity. Copyright of Silvia Bassini, 2024.

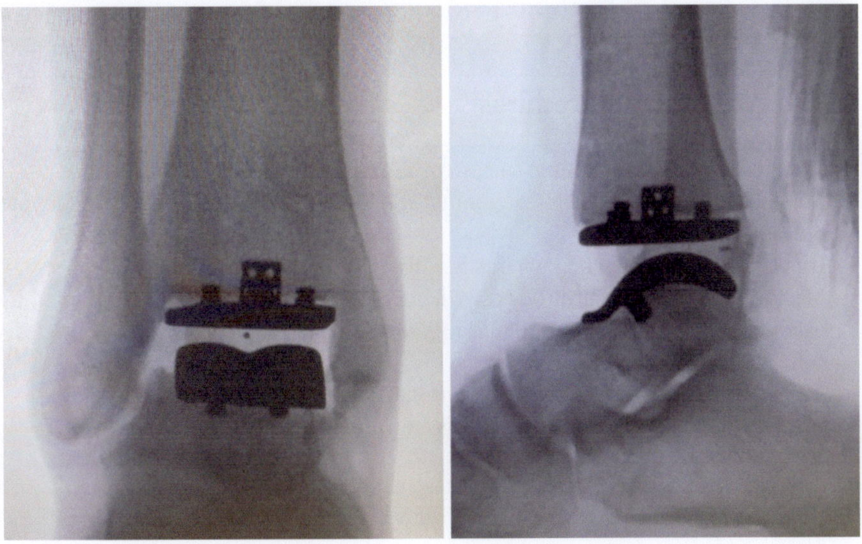

Fig. 19.4 Final postoperative X-ray showing an anterior approach TAR

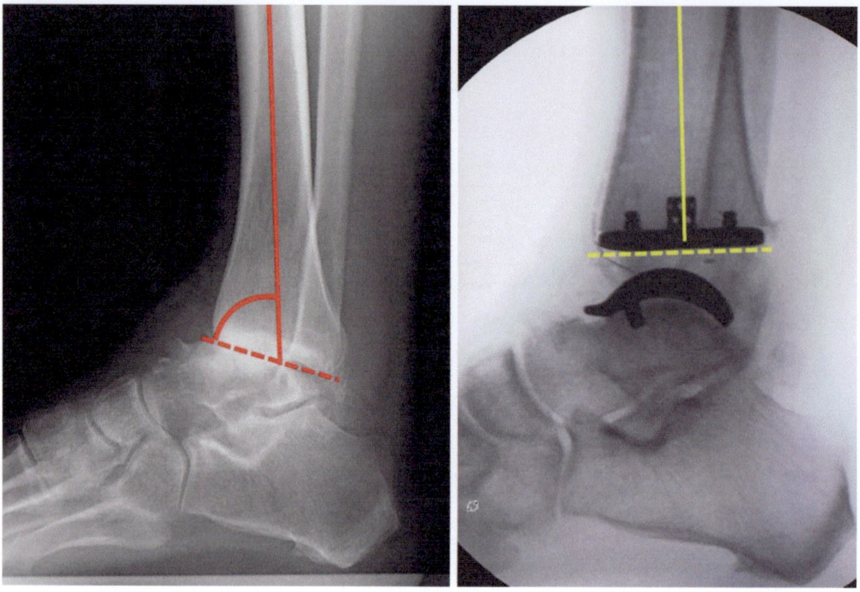

Fig. 19.5 Preoperative evidence of excessive distal tibial slope on the lateral view, associated to anteposition of the talar dome (at left); postoperative correction of the sagittal deformity with a slightly inverse tibial slope (at right)

19.4 Accessory Procedures

- Achilles tendon lengthening: in case of the Achilles tendon's retraction.
- Medial displaced calcaneal osteotomy: if valgus deformities of the hindfoot are present.
- Dwyer's osteotomy: when a varus hindfoot deformity is diagnosed.
- Midfoot and hindfoot arthrodesis: whether the joints of the foot are affected by osteoarthrosis, a fusion of subtalar joints, midtarsal joints, and triple arthrodesis can be conducted.
- Medial and lateral ligamentous repair: in case of instability of the ankle.
- Medial ligamentous release: if soft tissue varus is present.

19.5 Postoperative Care

Immediately after surgery, the patient is advised to wear a Walker boot for 3 weeks, ambulating with a partial weight-bearing. To allow plantarflexion and dorsiflexion to be performed actively and passively, the brace can be removed more times per day. During the fourth postoperative week, it is permissible to progressively get to ambulation with a full weight-bearing on the operated limb protected by a Walker boot. After 1 month from the implant of the prosthesis, no auxiliary aids are needed to walk.

There are some differences in postoperative treatment in the case of patients in whom ancillary bone procedures were required during surgery. Instead of the Walker boot, the operated ankle will be immobilized in a cast for 2 weeks without allowing weight-bearing on it. After 2 weeks, the cast is replaced by the orthopedic brace to be able to exercise flexion–extension of the ankle, but the weight-bearing is still not allowed till the fourth-week post-surgery when a partial load is permitted.

Take Home Messages

1. Ankle osteoarthritis is a common cause of disability, and total ankle replacement is a treatment whose indications are increasing, replacing, in different cases, arthrodesis.
2. The most common way to perform a TAR is via a direct anterior approach through the interval between the tibialis anterior and extensor hallucis longus tendons.
3. To properly plan a TAR, a physical examination, weight-bearing AP, and lateral X-ray of the ankle are needed.
4. Ancillary tools to be used in more complex cases can be: Salzman view X-ray, MRI, CT and SPECT-CT scan, and CAS.
5. Associated procedures are often necessary to fix extra- and intra-articular malignments in order to reduce overstress of the prosthetic components.

References

1. Valderrabano V, Horisberger M, Russell I, Dougall H, Hintermann B. Etiology of ankle osteoarthritis. Clin Orthop Relat Res. 2009;467(7):1800–6.
2. Mosca M, Caravelli S, Vocale E, et al. Clinical-radiological outcomes and complications after total ankle replacement through a lateral transfibular approach: a retrospective evaluation at a mid-term follow-up. Int Orthop. 2021;45(2):437–43.
3. Reb CW, Watson BC, Fidler CM, et al. Anterior ankle incision wound complications between Total ankle replacement and ankle arthrodesis: a matched cohort study. J Foot Ankle Surg. 2021;60(1):47–50.
4. Hintermann B, Ruiz R. Ankle arthritis and the treatment with ankle replacement. Rev Med Clin Condes. 2014;25(5):812–23.
5. Saltzman CL, el-Khoury GY. The hindfoot alignment view. Foot Ankle Int. 1995;16(9):572–6.
6. Choi WJ, Kim BS, Lee JW. Preoperative planning and surgical technique: how do I balance my ankle? Foot Ankle Int. 2012;33(3):244–9.
7. Farrier AJ, Ramaskandhan JR, Siddique MS, Green J. Preoperative templating in total ankle replacement – a case for 3D imaging. Foot Ankle Orthop. 2016;1(1) https://doi.org/10.1177/2473011416S00250. 2016 AOFAS Annual Meeting Abstracts.
8. Sun SP, Su HW. Full scale 3D preoperative planning system of the ankle joint replacement surgery with multimedia system. Smart Sci. 2014;2(2):80–4.
9. Mosca M, Caravelli S, Vocale E, et al. Clinical radiographical outcomes and complications after a brand-new total ankle replacement design through an anterior approach: a retrospective at a short-term follow up. J Clin Med. 2021;10(11):2258.
10. Usuelli FG, Maccario C, Indino C, Manzi L, Gross CE. Tibial slope in total ankle arthroplasty: anterior or lateral approach. Foot Ankle Surg. 2017;23(2):84–8.

Part VIII

Common Osteotomy Around Foot and Ankle in Adults

M. Mosca

Planning in Common Osteotomy Around Foot and Ankle in Adults

20

S. Caravelli, M. Viotto, M. Di Ponte, B. Khateeb, E. Vocale, G. Gardini, and M. Mosca

20.1 Introduction

Alterations of the hindfoot alignment are a cornerstone of orthopedic foot and ankle deformity correction [1]. Hindfoot and forefoot loading are influenced by the alignment of the hindfoot and calcaneal configuration; as part of the "tripod" of the foot, the position of the calcaneus is critically important to the alignment of the foot during weight-bearing [2].

A normal hindfoot alignment is defined when there is a hindfoot valgus angle of 0–5°, while an abnormal hindfoot alignment is defined as a hindfoot valgus angle greater than 10° or any degree of hindfoot varus [3]. The flatfoot, instead, is characterized by a triplanar deformity centered on the subtalar joint, resulting in a valgus malalignment of the hindfoot and a reduction of the medial plantar arch [4].

In the presence of symptomatic foot and ankle malalignment, a calcaneal osteotomy represents an important component in the restoration of hindfoot biomechanics [2]. Calcaneal osteotomies allow modification to the calcaneal axis, correction of its deformities, and a positive influence on walking dynamics across the various spatial planes [5].

Osteotomies through the calcaneus body not only realign the tuberosity but also redirect the pull of the Achilles tendon, making it a corrective rather than a deforming force [6]. Calcaneal osteotomies allow multiplane modification of the calcaneal axis and deformity correction, resulting in improved foot biomechanics [2].

Multiple calcaneal osteotomies have been described to address foot malalignment, incorporating numerous techniques to treat different pathologies that produce

S. Caravelli · M. Di Ponte · B. Khateeb · E. Vocale · G. Gardini · M. Mosca (✉)
Bentivoglio Orthopaedic Unit, IRCCS Istituto Ortopedico Rizzoli, Bologna, Italy
e-mail: massimiliano.mosca@ior.it

M. Viotto
IRCCS Istituto Ortopedico Rizzoli, S.C. Ortopedia Pediatria, Bologna, Italy

G. M. Marcheggiani Muccioli et al. (eds.), *Easy Planning in Elective Primary Orthopedic Procedures*, https://doi.org/10.1007/978-3-031-77006-7_20

varus and valgus hindfoot deformity [2, 7, 8]. Most commonly, the medial displacement calcaneal osteotomy (MDCO) and the lateral column lengthening (LCL) are used for the treatment of different types of pes planovalgus [7], while a lateral closing wedge, or the Dwyer's osteotomy, is used for the treatment of pes cavovarus [8].

20.2 Clinical and Imaging Assessment

The *physical exam* should consist mainly of inspection, palpation, evaluation of the range of motion (ROM), testing the muscle strength, and gait analysis. Both feet should be evaluated to allow a comparison between the affected limb and the contralateral one. The various tests and valuations should be performed with the patient in a supine position and standing to understand properly how the feet change with weight-bearing.

In the case of cavovarus foot, the Coleman–Andreasi "block test" is a critical portion of the examination as one of the major goals of the physical exam is to determine the rigidity of the deformity. This test should be performed to understand if the varus hindfoot is correctable. The examinator asks the patient to stand on a hindfoot support or "block" high enough to avoid the forefoot touching the ground when placing the plantar-flexed first metatarsal over the block's edge. The metatarsals are put off the edge while the hindfoot remains on the block. This way, the plantar-flexed first metatarsal cannot tilt the foot into the varus. If the hindfoot varus remains, then the deformity is fixed. However, if the hindfoot corrects to physiologic valgus, then the deformity is flexible and driven by the forefoot deformity [9].

Hindfoot varus is confirmed through the "peek-a-boo" heel sign, which is the clinical condition whereby the heel is visible on the medial side when viewing the patient from the front with the feet in neutral rotation [10].

Imaging diagnosis is based on weight-bearing dorso-plantar and lateral *conventional radiographs* (CR). In addition to these, both Cobey's and Buck's techniques are classic and popular hindfoot alignment assessment methods. To obtain a proper Cobey radiograph, the X-ray beam needs to be oriented to tilt 20° with the horizontal plane to emit behind the feet and focus on the heel; the X-ray detector needs to be oriented to tilt 20° with the vertical plane and placed in front of the feet; the X-ray beam needs to be kept perpendicular to the detector; the subjects must stand on a radiolucent platform with equal weight on both feet facing the detector with the medial border of their feet parallel and about 10 cm apart; and the X-ray tube has to be positioned approximately 1 m away from the heel. The Buck technique is the same, but with the detector positioned vertically so that in this way better images could be acquired quicker with easier operation [11]. In 1995, Saltzman modified Cobey's technique to illuminate the normative data for the radiographic alignment of the tibia and calcaneus, and the technique is often known as Saltzman's view today [12].

Since *magnetic resonance* (MR) images are acquired under non-weight-bearing conditions, they are not yet considered to be reliable for quantification of hindfoot alignment. However, the medial and lateral contours of the calcaneus and the sustentaculum tali, visible in the coronal plane of a T1-weighted MR, are anatomical landmarks useful for measuring the hindfoot alignment. Studies showed how the medial calcaneal contour allows the highest accuracy to detect a hindfoot valgus, while for the hindfoot valgus the highest accuracy for detection is reached using the sustentaculum tangent. Even if these results can allow a suspect of an alteration of the hindfoot alignment, there was no perfect correlation to measurements on radiographs [3].

Since the MR is not the first tool a doctor can use to diagnose an alteration of the hindfoot, radiologists could have a relative lack of awareness of hindfoot malalignment on ankle MR; according to this, a review of reports of ankle MRI studies by consultant musculoskeletal radiologists reporting for a Foot and Ankle Unit specialist has shown a significant underreporting of hindfoot valgus [13].

Newer *magnetic resonance imaging* modalities, such as T2 mapping techniques, have also been tested for early diagnosis of osteoarthritis (OA), although these techniques have proven more useful in assessing before surgery [14].

As previously reported, the imaging diagnosis is based on weight-bearing X-rays [11]. However, all hindfoot alignment measurements based on standard radiographs impose a substantial risk for measurement errors due to malpositioning, inconsistent angulation, or enlargement of foot and ankle skeletal structures caused by the radiographic fan beam. In more recent years, the appearance and development of the weight-bearing computer tomography (WB-CT) scan has allowed a better 3D understanding of defects of bone segmentation and OA, associated supra- and inframalleolar deformities of the foot and ankle, in a physiological, standing, and loaded condition and eventually could help overcome some of the measurement errors of the X-rays [15, 16, 17].

There are different methods to determine hindfoot alignment on weight-bearing CT, including the use of the medial calcaneal border and the hindfoot angle that Burssens et al. proposed, which includes both talus and calcaneum. The talar shift on which the angle is based can aid the surgeon preoperatively in determining how much translation is necessary to obtain a neutral alignment during a calcaneal osteotomy. In addition to a weight-bearing CT, it is advised to add a full leg view when a clinical bowing is noted, or supra—malleolar malalignment is suspected [15]. An additional reason to get a CT is the Torque Ankle Lever Arm System (TALAS), a software algorithm on WB-CT scans based on an inverted three-dimensional (3D) pyramid model, which has been validated as a reliable and reproducible semiautomatic tool for measuring hindfoot alignment. The algorithm calculates foot ankle offset (FAO), calcaneal offset (CO), and hindfoot angle (HA) [17].

20.3 Calcaneal Osteotomies for Correction of Planovalgus Foot

Koutsogiannis et al. described a medial and plantar translation through an oblique osteotomy of the posterior calcaneal tuberosity. This technique has evolved to what is recognized today as the MDCO [18].

The concept of modifying the "external column" was presented by Evans, who described the effect of lateral column length alteration on the control of midfoot abduction and adduction and presented the lateral column lengthening osteotomy, now known as Evans' osteotomy [19].

Over the years, these two techniques of double coronal–axial plane osteotomy remain the workhorse of hindfoot valgus correction [2].

20.3.1 Operative Techniques

In both cases, the patient is positioned in a lateral decubitus position on the healthy side to be able to perform the surgical approach comfortably, considering anatomical references and reducing surgical time.

The classic surgical approach to *MDCO* is through an oblique lateral incision, determined by using a reference point that is one-third of the distance from the tip of the lateral malleolus to the posteroinferior margin of the calcaneus, saving the sural nerve [20].

The lateral calcaneus cortex is exposed, and the osteotomy is performed using an oscillating saw. The osteotomy technique includes cutting of the lateral, dorsal, and plantar cortices. The posterior osteotomy fragment is manually mobilized and shifted medially, 7–15 mm medially. The authors of this brief chapter prefer to use Kirschner wires (KW) to fix the osteotomy, such as a Kapandji technique, holding the sliding correction. Eventually, the positioning of the KW is checked by fluoroscopy (the Kirschner wire should not trespass the subtalar articular surface). Once

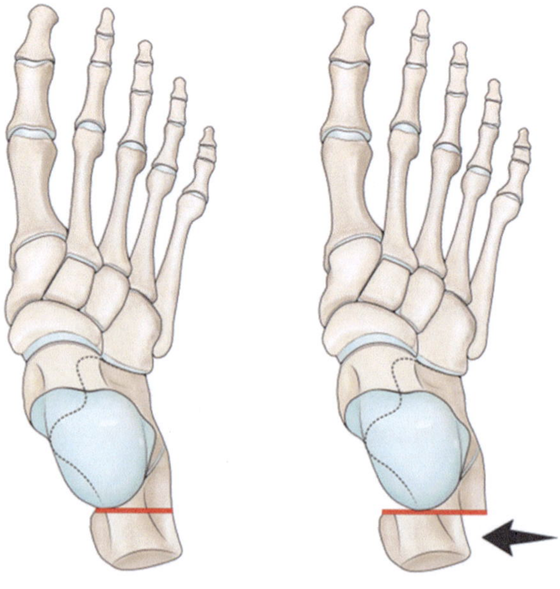

Fig. 20.1 Medial displacement calcaneal osteotomy. In evidence the posterior tuberosity sliding in a dorso-plantar view. Copyright of Silvia Bassini, 2024. All rights reserved

we are satisfied with the shifting and position, the osteotomy can be stabilized with two cannulated compression screws (Fig. 20.1).

In case of *Evans procedure*, the position on the operating table is the same as MDCO. An oblique skin incision approximately 4 cm in length is made over the lateral aspect of the calcaneus, centered over the site of osteotomy. Incisional landmarks include the anterior apophysis of the calcaneus distally and the inferior surface of the calcaneus proximally.

Dissection is deepened through the subcutaneous tissue, taking care of the superficial crossing veins; the subcutaneous tissue is elevated from the surface of the deep fascia in a circumferential manner to expose the majority of the extensor digitorum muscle belly (EDB). The peroneal tendons are retracted plantarly. With reflection of the extensor digitorum muscle belly superiorly and the peroneal tendons inferiorly, the lateral aspect of the calcaneus is exposed. Next, the calcaneal–cuboid joint is identified. The osteotomy must be made parallel to the calcaneal–cuboid joint. Once the obliquity of the joint is visualized, a periosteal incision is made approximately 1 cm proximal and parallel to the calcaneal–cuboid joint. The periosteum is specifically left intact distally as to avoid disruption of the dorsal calcaneal–cuboid joint ligaments. At this point, a sagittal saw is used to cut the calcaneal osteotomy. The osteotomy is made approximately 1 cm proximal and parallel to the calcaneal–cuboid joint. The medial cortex of the calcaneus is contacted but not transected, creating a stable hinge for distracting the osteotomy. An Hintermann retractor is positioned to distract the osteotomy approximately 1 cm, and the range of motion of the subtalar and midtarsal joints is evaluated (Fig. 20.2).

With both manual manipulation and intraoperative fluoroscopy, a bone graft was then fashioned to press-fit the open defect of the calcaneus. The distractor is then removed. If the osteotomy and graft are stable, no internal fixation device has been

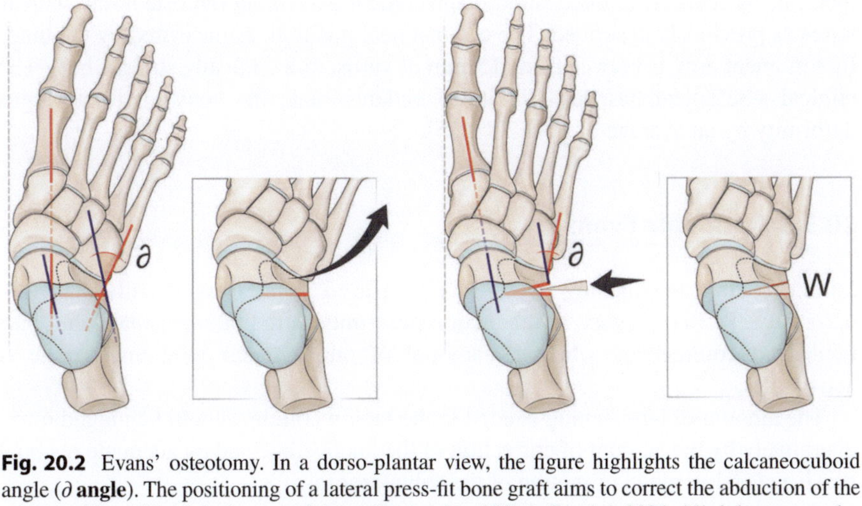

Fig. 20.2 Evans' osteotomy. In a dorso-plantar view, the figure highlights the calcaneocuboid angle (∂ **angle**). The positioning of a lateral press-fit bone graft aims to correct the abduction of the midfoot. **W**: width of the bone graft base. Copyright of Silvia Bassini, 2024. All rights reserved

found to be necessary. The final outcome is then reassessed by clinical manipulation and intraoperative fluoroscopy.

20.3.2 Rationale MDCO

The MDCO shifts the mechanical axis of the calcaneus from a more lateral position to a more medial position. This also shifts the action of the Achilles tendon medially, which minimizes the everting deforming effect and improves the inversion forces. The clinical goal of the hindfoot valgus correction is to achieve a clinically neutral heel, as defined by a vertical axis from the heel up to the longitudinal axis of the Achilles tendon and distal aspect of the leg [21].

20.3.2.1 Planning

First, the hindfoot alignment angle (HAA), formed by the intersection of the longitudinal axis of the tibial shaft and the axis of the calcaneal tuberosity (normal angle, 5.6 ± 5.4°; flatfoot deformity, 22.5 ± 4.9°), is measured to make the diagnosis of flatfoot [22].

Hindfoot valgus can be better evaluated on a hindfoot alignment view radiograph by measuring the distance between the weight-bearing axis of the tibia and the most inferior aspect of the calcaneus, which has been defined as the hindfoot moment arm (HMA) [23].

Chan et al. derived a linear regression mode for the MDCO in relation to the change in the hindfoot moment arm, demonstrating that a medial translation of 1 mm corresponds to approximately a 1.52-mm change in radiographic HMA [24].

Using a calibrated X-ray, it is possible, through the analysis of the HMA expressed in millimeters, to plan the amount of shift. The desired displacement can be obtained by using a dedicated plate, which allows different measures of displacement, or by measuring the desired displacement and fixing the osteotomy with K wires as previously described. The optimal heel position, as measured by the hindfoot moment arm, is between 0 and 5 mm of varus, or a clinically straight heel. The clinical assessment has been shown to underestimate the bony hindfoot valgus deformity by an average of 11–12.8° [25].

20.3.3 Rationale Evans

Lateral column lengthening (LCL) has been used in progressive collapsing foot deformity (PCFD) surgery for abduction deformity at the talonavicular joint, particularly recommended when the amount of talonavicular joint uncoverage is above 40%.

The amount of lengthening needed in the lateral column should be judged intraoperatively by the amount of correction of the uncoverage and by adequate residual passive eversion range of motion of the subtalar joint.

Performing the correct amount of lengthening is a critical portion of the operation. The amount will vary for each case, but the range of ideal graft size was 5–10 mm. A pin distractor can be placed across the osteotomy and opened gradually to allow for correction of the forefoot abduction. The ideal amount of correction is assessed both visually and with a simulated AP weight-bearing fluoroscopic view.

Overcorrection will lead to a higher rate of lateral column pain and increased lateral foot pressures with a higher rate of patient dissatisfaction [26].

20.3.3.1 Planning

We measured the TFA and calcaneocuboid angle (CCA) using a software program for planning foot and ankle osteotomy. The correction was achieved when the foot was hinged on the medial calcaneal cortex and rotated on the center of the imaginary circle of the talar head until the TFA was 0 or collinear. Performing this maneuver created an opening wedge in the anterior neck of the calcaneus, which corresponded to the proposed graft size. The lateral cortical margin of the calcaneus was measured to determine the length (in mm) of the base of the Evans wedge graft [27].

To fill the gap, there are three possibilities: the use of a pre-shaped allograft wedge, the use of an autograft wedge, or the use of trabecular metal wedges with usually three different standard sizes.

20.4 Calcaneal Osteotomies for Correction of Cavovarus

Multiple calcaneal osteotomies have been described for the treatment of cavovarus [28]. *Dwyer's osteotomy* is considered the more classic lateral shifting osteotomy of the calcaneus, achieved by a lateral closing wedge osteotomy of the posterior tuberosity [9].

20.4.1 Technique

The patient is positioned in a lateral decubitus position on the healthy side to be able to perform the surgical approach comfortably, considering anatomical references. The approach to the calcaneus is through a lateral oblique skin incision posteriorly and inferiorly to the peroneal tendons, directly to the lateral aspect of the calcaneal tuberosity, such as the MDCO.

The lateral calcaneus cortex is exposed, and the osteotomy is performed through an oscillating saw. The osteotomy technique includes cutting of the lateral, dorsal, and plantar cortices. The medial cortex of the calcaneus is contacted and to protect the medial neurovascular bundle, an osteotome to complete the osteotomy is recommended.

Laterally based wedge is removed by subtracting a 1 cm base lateral wedge. The posterior osteotomy fragment is manually mobilized to close the gap, performing a closing wedge osteotomy. If the correction is not enough, it can be associated with a lateral slide of the posterior tuberosity. The osteotomy is stabilized with two cannulated screws under fluoroscopy control. Clinical assessment of the subtalar joint range of motion and peroneal tendons tightness also needs to be done.

20.4.2 Rationale Dwyer

The resection of an adequate wedge of bone realigns the calcaneal tuberosity lateral to the weight-bearing line of the tibia; this could prevent the recurrence of deformity. Dwyer calcaneal osteotomy also allows the Achilles tendon to become a corrective force instead of a deforming force because the calcaneus is no longer in varus [29].

20.4.2.1 Planning

Two reference lines are drawn to determine the level and the amount of the calcaneal osteotomy: a proximal one (tibial anatomic axis) and a distal one (calcaneal bisection). A third one, the distal reference line, is marked 10 mm medial and parallel to the calcaneal bisection line. The point in the calcaneal body, at the intersection between the proximal and distal normal reference lines, is where the center of rotation angulation (CORA) is placed. Once the CORA is identified, a wedge can be removed to realign the calcaneus to a vertical position (parallel to the proximal reference line). The first K wire and the subsequent osteotomy are perpendicular to the tibia anatomic axis. The second K wire and the subsequent osteotomy are perpendicular to the distal reference line. The lateral cortical margin of the calcaneus was measured to determine the length (in mm) of the base of the wedge. It is possible that even after this procedure, the calcaneus remains medially displaced from the anatomical axis of the tibia; in these cases, the tuberosity should be translated laterally, breaking the medial cortical hinge with an osteotome (Fig. 20.3) [29].

Take Home Messages

1. Hindfoot deformities can represent a common cause of pain and disability.
2. Calcaneal osteotomies are considered important tools to deal with hindfoot malalignment nowadays. Medial displacement calcaneal osteotomy, Evans' osteotomy, and Dwyer's osteotomy are the most common procedures.
3. To properly plan a calcaneal osteotomy, weight-bearing dorso-plantar and lateral X-ray of the foot and Saltzmann view are needed.
4. Correct planning and the proper position of the patient during the surgery are needed to choose the right correction entity wisely.

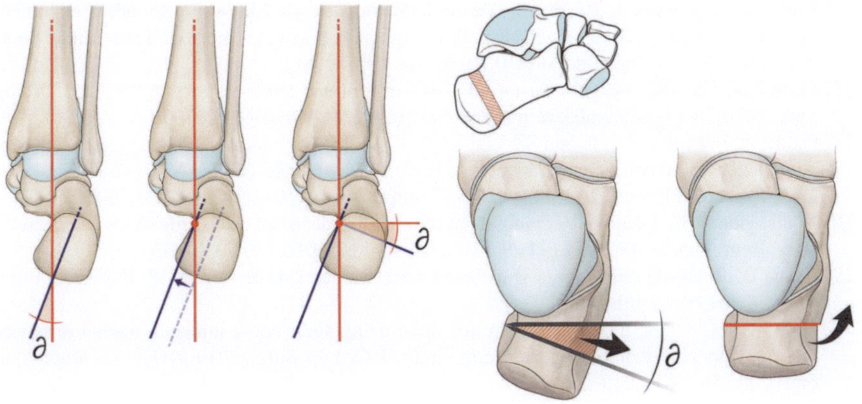

Fig. 20.3 Dwyer calcaneal osteotomy. Copyright of Silvia Bassini, 2024. All rights reserved

References

1. Prat D, Lee W, Farber DC. Calcaneal osteotomies. Ann Jt. 2020;5:29. https://doi.org/10.21037/aoj.2020.02.02.
2. Tennant JN, Carmont M, Phisitkul P. Calcaneus osteotomy. Curr Rev Musculoskelet Med. 2014;7(4):271–6. https://doi.org/10.1007/s12178-014-9237-8.
3. Buck FM, et al. Diagnostic performance of MRI measurements to assess hindfoot malalignment. An assessment of four measurement techniques. Eur Radiol. 2013;23(9):2594–601. https://doi.org/10.1007/s00330-013-2839-5.
4. Lee MS, et al. Diagnosis and treatment of adult flatfoot. Foot Ankle Surg. 2005;44(2):78–113. https://doi.org/10.1053/j.jfas.2004.12.001.
5. Malerba F, De Marchi F. Calcaneal osteotomies. Foot Ankle Clin. 2005;10(3):523–40. https://doi.org/10.1016/j.fcl.2005.04.005.
6. Huber H, Galantay R, Dutoit M. Avascular necrosis after osteotomy of the talar neck to correct residual club-foot deformity in children. A long-term review. J Bone Joint Surg Br. 2002;84(3):426–30. https://doi.org/10.1302/0301-620x.84b3.12206.
7. Tao X, Chen W, Tang K. Surgical procedures for treatment of adult acquired flatfoot deformity: a network meta-analysis. J Orthop Surg. 2019;14(1):62. https://doi.org/10.1186/s13018-019-1094-0.
8. Dwyer FC. Osteotomy of the calcaneum for pes cavus. J Bone Joint Surg Br. 1959;41-B(1):80–6. https://doi.org/10.1302/0301-620X.41B1.80.
9. Foran IM, et al. Impact of coleman block test on adult hindfoot alignment assessed by clinical examination, radiography, and weight-bearing computed tomography. Foot Ankle Orthop. 2020;5(3):2473011420933264. https://doi.org/10.1177/2473011420933264.
10. Maynou C, Szymanski C, Thiounn A. The adult cavus foot. EFORT Open Rev. 2017;2(5):221–9. https://doi.org/10.1302/2058-5241.2.160077.
11. Yang C, Xu X, Hu M, Wang B, Zhu Y, Liu J. Optimization of hindfoot alignment radiography. Acta Radiol. 2017;58(6):719–25. https://doi.org/10.1177/0284185116668214.
12. Saltzman CL, el-Khoury GY. The hindfoot alignment view. Foot Ankle Int. 1995;16(9):572–6. https://doi.org/10.1177/107110079501600911.
13. Junaid SE, et al. The awareness of hindfoot malalignment on non-weight-bearing ankle MRI. Skeletal Radiol. 2021;50(7):1317–23. https://doi.org/10.1007/s00256-020-03674-8.
14. Schreiner MM, et al. New technology in imaging cartilage of the ankle. Cartilage. 2017;8(1):31–41. https://doi.org/10.1177/1947603516632848.

15. Burssens A, Peeters J, Buedts K, Victor J, Vandeputte G. Measuring hindfoot alignment in weight bearing CT: a novel clinical relevant measurement method. Foot Ankle Surg. 2016;22(4):233–8. https://doi.org/10.1016/j.fas.2015.10.002.
16. Conti MS, Ellis SJ. Weight-bearing CT scans in foot and ankle surgery. J Am Acad Orthop Surg. 2020;28(14):e595–603. https://doi.org/10.5435/JAAOS-D-19-00700.
17. Haldar A, Bernasconi A, Junaid SE, Lee KHB, Welck M, Saifuddin A. 3D imaging for hindfoot alignment assessment: a comparative study between non-weight-bearing MRI and weight-bearing CT. Skeletal Radiol. 2021;50(1):179–88. https://doi.org/10.1007/s00256-020-03532-7.
18. Koutsogiannis E. Treatment of mobile flat foot by displacement osteotomy of the calcaneus. J Bone Joint Surg Br. 1971;53-B(1):96–100. https://doi.org/10.1302/0301-620x.53b1.96.
19. Evans D. Relapsed club foot. J Bone Joint Surg Br. 1961;43-B(4):722–33. https://doi.org/10.1302/0301-620X.43B4.722.
20. Park J-H, et al. The incision strategy for minimizing sural nerve injury in medial displacement calcaneal osteotomy: a cadaveric study. J Orthop Surg. 2019;14(1):356. https://doi.org/10.1186/s13018-019-1411-7.
21. Schon LC, et al. Consensus for the indication of a medializing displacement calcaneal osteotomy in the treatment of progressive collapsing foot deformity. Foot Ankle Int. 2020;41(10):1282–5. https://doi.org/10.1177/1071100720950747.
22. Cody EA, Williamson ER, Burket JC, Deland JT, Ellis SJ. Correlation of talar anatomy and subtalar joint alignment on weightbearing computed tomography with radiographic flatfoot parameters. Foot Ankle Int. 2016;37(8):874–81. https://doi.org/10.1177/1071100716646629.
23. Conti MS, Garfinkel JH, Ellis SJ. Outcomes of reconstruction of the flexible adult-acquired flatfoot deformity. Orthop Clin North Am. 2020;51(1):109–20. https://doi.org/10.1016/j.ocl.2019.08.005.
24. Chan JY, et al. The contribution of medializing calcaneal osteotomy on hindfoot alignment in the reconstruction of the stage II adult acquired flatfoot deformity. Foot Ankle Int. 2013;34(2):159–66. https://doi.org/10.1177/1071100712460225.
25. de Cesar Netto C, Kunas GC, Soukup D, Marinescu A, Ellis SJ. Correlation of clinical evaluation and radiographic hindfoot alignment in stage II adult-acquired flatfoot deformity. Foot Ankle Int. 2018;39(7):771–9. https://doi.org/10.1177/1071100718762113.
26. Thordarson DB, et al. Consensus for the indication of lateral column lengthening in the treatment of progressive collapsing foot deformity. Foot Ankle Int. 2020;41(10):1286–8. https://doi.org/10.1177/1071100720950732.
27. Siddiqui NA, Lamm BM. Digital planning for foot and ankle deformity correction: Evans osteotomy. Foot Ankle Surg. 2014;53(6):700–5. https://doi.org/10.1053/j.jfas.2014.04.011.
28. Bariteau JT, Blankenhorn BD, Tofte JN, DiGiovanni CW. What is the role and limit of calcaneal osteotomy in the cavovarus foot? Foot Ankle Clin. 2013;18(4):697–714. https://doi.org/10.1016/j.fcl.2013.08.001.
29. Lamm BM, Gesheff MG, Salton HL, Dupuis TW, Zeni F. Preoperative planning and intraoperative technique for accurate realignment of the Dwyer calcaneal osteotomy. Foot Ankle Surg. 2012;51(6):743–8. https://doi.org/10.1053/j.jfas.2012.08.004.

MIX
Papier aus verantwortungsvollen Quellen
Paper from responsible sources
FSC® C105338

If you have any concerns about our products,
you can contact us on
ProductSafety@springernature.com

In case Publisher is established outside the EU,
the EU authorized representative is:
Springer Nature Customer Service Center GmbH
Europaplatz 3, 69115 Heidelberg, Germany

Printed by Libri Plureos GmbH
in Hamburg, Germany